# Managed Care Networks:
# Principles and practice

# Managed Care Networks:
## Principles and practice

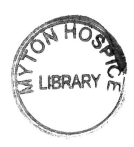

*Edited by*

Roger James MRCP FRCR
*Clinical Director of Cancer Services, Kent Cancer Network, Oncology Department,*
*Mid-Kent NHS Trust, Maidstone, Kent*

Andrew Miles MSc MPhil PhD
*Professor of Public Health Policy and Editor-in-Chief,*
Journal of Evaluation in Clinical Practice, *University of East London, UK*

UeL University Centre for
Public Health Policy &
Health Services Research

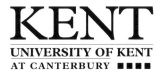

AESCULAPIUS MEDICAL PRESS
LONDON  SAN FRANCISCO  SYDNEY

Published by

Aesculapius Medical Press (London, San Francisco, Sydney)
Centre for Public Health Policy and Health Services Research
School of Health Sciences
University of East London
PO Box LB48, London EC1A 1LB


© Aesculapius Medical Press 2002

First published 2002

**British Library Cataloguing in Publication Data**
A catalogue record for this book is available from the British Library

ISBN 1 903044 27 8

While the advice and information in this book are believed to be true and accurate at the
time of going to press, neither the authors nor the publishers nor the sponsoring institutions
can accept any legal responsibility or liability for any errors or omissions that may be made.
In particular (but without limiting the generality of the preceding disclaimer) every effort
has been made to check drug usages; however, it is possible that errors have been missed.
Furthermore, dosage schedules are constantly being revised and new side effects recognised.
For these reasons, the reader is strongly urged to consult the drug companies' printed
instructions before administering any of the drugs recommended in this book.

*Further copies of this volume are available from:*
Claudio Melchiorri
Research Dissemination Fellow
Centre for Public Health Policy and Health Services Research
School of Health Sciences
University of East London
PO Box LB48, London EC1A 1LB

Fax: 020 8525 8661
email: claudio@keyadvances4.demon.co.uk


Typeset, printed and bound in Britain
Peter Powell Origination and Print Limited

# Contents

# Contributors

William Audeh MD, Associate Chief Medical Officer, Salick Health Care, Inc., Los Angeles, California, USA

Roger Cooley PhD, Lecturer, Computing Laboratory, University of Kent at Canterbury

Ewan Ferlie BA PhD, Professor of Public Service Management, Management School, Imperial College of Science, Technology and Medicine, London

Jane M Gillies PhD, Cranfield School of Management, Cranfield University, Cranfield, UK

Chris Hawkins BA MA MCSP SRP, Fellow, Centre for Creativity, Strategy and Change, Warwick Business School, University of Warwick

Roger James MRCP FRCR, Clinical Director of Cancer Services, Kent Cancer Network, Oncology Department, Mid-Kent NHS Trust, Maidstone, Kent

Beth Kewell BA PhD, Senior Lecturer in Organisation Studies, Bristol Business School, University of the West of England

Ian P McCarthy PhD, Principal Fellow, Organisational Systems and Strategy Unit, International Manufacturing Centre, University of Warwick, Coventry

Roderick Neame MB BChir MA PhD, Chief Executive, Health Information Consulting Ltd, Faversham, Kent

James W Rimmer BSc MSc, ASWCS Programme Director, Avon, Somerset & Wiltshire Cancer Services, Bristol

Beverley Salt, Marketing Company President, AstraZeneca UK Ltd, Kings Langley, Herts

Peter Spurgeon BSc(Hons) PhD ABPS, Professor of Health Services Management & Director of Management/Organisational Development & Leadership, Health Services Management Centre, Edgbaston, Birmingham

Liz Watson BSc MSc, Executive Director of Strategy & Performance Management, North Staffordshire Health Authority, Stoke-on-Trent, Staffordshire

Tera Younger MSc, Independent Health Consultant, London

# Preface

The future management of cancer, cardiology, emergency services and mental health in the UK is set to occur within the context of managed care networks, but little has been published on their conceptual and methodological framework. If this is to be a British phenomenon, where is the guidance for those British managers and clinicians who are charged with their construction, operation and maintenance? Are there any models that might make the phenomenon more accessible? How do we change an organisation based on institutions into one based on diseases (cancer, cardiac, diabetes) or hospital departments (accident and emergency departments or emergency rooms)? Do we have the technology to enable an individual patient to access his or her health record across the variety of institutions? The present volume aims to address these questions through a systematic treatment of the principles and practices of care networks.

UK Public Sector Networks are likely to increase in importance through the twenty-first century. A series of health policies operate across health, education and social welfare sectors. Most British deaths are caused by smoking and unhealthy eating, which starts in childhood. Teenage smoking and 'junk foods' are linked with deprivation, school truancy and criminalisation. But not all cross-sector problems are as long term as this. Hospital accident and emergency department trolley waits are linked to hospital ward 'bed blocking', in turn caused by inconsistencies in provision of independent sector accommodation for elderly people. These sorts of issues are being tackled by Public Sector Agreements (PSAs), led through local authority Scrutiny Committees, which bring together police, social services and education experts to tackle what used to be called 'public health problems'. The population served by PSAs needs to be formalised and regulated to avoid boundary duplications.

Professors Ferlie and Spurgeon, in the first two chapters, point to some of the forces driving care networks in the NHS. Over the last 10 years a series of issues have raised concern. The UK has some of the worst survival rates for the common diseases of the 'civilised' world, such as heart attacks, stroke and cancer. UK annual expenditure on health per capita is inferior to that of many countries with much smaller gross domestic products.

The year 2000 saw the most dramatic changes in the NHS since its inception 55 years previously. Networks were introduced at the same time as major changes in the primary sector. Primary care organisations (PCOs) collate community and general practice health care. They receive all NHS development funding direct from the Department of Health and commission services for their local health economy, which usually contains a district general hospital. However, the future of this venerable institution is also in the balance. The last years of the century saw a rash of hospital 'mergers' or 'closures'. A conference organised by the Eastern Regional Office in June 2001 questioned the validity of local hospital-based acute services in the context of the development of PCOs (NHS Eastern Regional Office 2001).

In her chapter on the role of pharmaceutical companies in managed networks, Beverly Salt reminds us of the long relationship between the industry and the NHS. Many world leaders, such as ICI, Wellcome and Pfizer, emerged as suppliers of agricultural products during the days of the Empire. Their successors, such as AstraZeneca, are strong enough to maintain a British stamp despite mergers and remain major foreign exchange earners for the UK. They contribute to the pre-eminence of the London Stock Exchange and British health research. Most doctors feel that better drugs will be the key to the improving UK survival rates and they see the genome project as providing a revolutionary approach to their design. Newly licensed drugs are promoted freely across the world. However, in the UK their uptake appears to many doctors to be hampered rather than expedited by the deliberations of the National Institute for Clinical Excellence (NICE). Cost as well as effectiveness are evaluated by NICE and some doctors suspect that the Treasury may well be looking with anxiety over the Atlantic. As Bill Audeh points out in his chapter on Salick Health Care, the USA annual inflation on cancer drugs is running at 35%, giving annual bills around $US200 billion. The NHS could respond only by increasing general taxation. One alternative might be to follow the French model: seek cross-party consensus using a 'Cancer Care Bill'.

The two chapters on cancer networks take up the theme of differences between tax-based and insurance-based health systems. The NHS covers the total UK population and appears to be spending half per capita of what is spent in the USA. Access is straightforward, the GP remains the gatekeeper to the secondary sector, and the uptake for screening and immunisation is 30% higher than in the USA. Most of the 34 English cancer networks are co-terminal with the new strategic health authorities and with local authority (county council) boundaries and they will co-ordinate commissioning from 7 to 10 PCOs. However, it is not clear what the role of the PCT will be in commissioning.

However, the NHS is performing poorly on a series of USA health priorities. Apart from our miserable survival rates for common 'Westernised' diseases, we have inferior electronic linkage, evidence or protocol-based practice and skill-mix utilisation. Furthermore, there is no financial incentive in the NHS for clinicians to excel or get involved in budgeting. However, there are important similarities between the two systems. Both have moved resources into primary care and are attempting to weed out poor practice by evidence-based regulation. Health maintenance organisations (HMOs) in the USA commission network care in the same way as we expect NHS PCOs to commission NHS networks. Both health systems emphasise the personal responsibility of the individual for his or her health and social care.

James Rimmer picks up a point made by Ewan Ferlie: it appears that implementation of the ground-breaking Calman–Hine Report (1995), recommending reorganisation of cancer services, has been patchy, incoherent and incomplete. However, in the last 2 years, things have been moving fast. Phase 1 of the Cancer Services Collaborative was started in 1999. The Cancer Czar, Professor Mike Richards, was appointed in 2000 and by the year end had published *The National Cancer Plan*. In April 2001, all

English cancer services were rearranged into 34 networks and accredited by peer review (using standards derived from the Calman–Hine Report) within 9 months. Most cancer networks have boundaries defined by the catchment area for a radiotherapy department and are co-terminal with the 28 new strategic health authorities. By the end of 2001, three network lead posts had been appointed in each network (their 102 names are available from the National Cancer Action Team in St Thomas' Hospital, London). By April 2002 each network will have published a 3-year Service Development Plan (SDP) to take advantage of an extra £570 million announced by Ministers in 2001. The SDP is required to establish local (network) machinery for cancer prevention (reducing smoking and junk foods), an extension of breast screening into an older age group, population-based reconfiguration of rarer cancers and a clear plan for workforce development.

In the final section of the book, Jane Gillies and Ian McCarthy echo Ewan Ferlie's warning that centralised, regulatory management is by far the most serious challenge to the emerging networks. The Department of Health is collecting returns on what appears to be an infinite series of access targets covering the time from referral to first outpatient appointment to diagnosis, and to treatment. By 2005 Ministers expect any patient with cancer to be treated within a month of diagnosis. NHS cancer targets are now as important to hospital chief executives as trolley or 18-month waits.

A good example of conflicting centralised policies is seen in the NHS cancer networks. The '2-week' wait policy for cancer requires all patients suspected by their GP of having cancer to be seen in hospital within 2 weeks of referral. It has improved cancer services, but the hit rate of the 'rapid access clinics' is only 20–30%. This means that the capacity of scarce hospital diagnostic services is occupied by large numbers of anxious people, very few of whom actually have cancer. The 2-week wait policy has in effect implemented a cancer screening service with no extra funding or plans to assess its cost-effectiveness. However, because of the nature of the disease, most patients with cancer are not suspected either by themselves or by their GPs of having it. Although the 2-week wait 'walking well' are being reassured by rapid access bronchoscopy, endoscopy and scanning, patients with undiagnosed cancers are sitting on wards awaiting the same tests. Hospital chief executives are asking why their beds are blocked. Clinicians required to treat non-cancer patients point to a policy that prolongs waiting times for non-cancer-related diagnostic tests.

Gillies and McCarthy emphasise that centralised, regulatory management frameworks are intuitively damaging to networks, which are seeking a 'third way'. This lies between the jungle of blame-directed, league-tabled competition and the rock face of the old-style NHS. The third way deals effectively with a rapidly changing, unpredictable yet innovative health industry. It requires a sharing of common values, resources and knowledge. As Professor Ferlie points out, network management style is diplomatic rather than hierarchical or entrepreneurial. If it is to achieve its goals, ministers need to clarify what they mean by network management, commissioning, data collection and accountability.

The final three chapters point out the essential links between data collection, accountability and governance in networks. Outcome data underpin both clinical governance and accountability in managed networks. Terra Younger sets out a working model for the accountability of networks. Roddy Neame recommends a web-based solution to make it run and this point is echoed in the final chapter in which Roger Cooley and Roger James point to the weekly multidisciplinary team meeting as the nodal point for all three functions in cancer networks.

English cancer doctors have been urgently requesting the facilities to collect reliable data on the impact of cancer services on outcomes and Scottish Health Networks have developed impressive guidelines for this methodology. Doctors are delighted that the national cancer minimum data-set (NCMDS) will be implemented from April 2002. However, they caution against repeating cancer registration problems identified by the Gillis report (2000). As Neame and James and Cooley point out, the NCMDS should be collected in real time. It will need modern electronic technology that allows cross-institutional data transfer by clinicians monitoring their own performance. However, this sort of technology is not a priority for the institutional-based national electronic patient record (EPR) programme and is not required to deliver cancer priorities such as electronic prescribing until 2004. The 'LIS' community governs EPR systems procurement and is committed to wiring institutions rather than connecting them together into networks. Once again, some department-directed top-slicing may be the answer.

At a public meeting in 2001 the Chief Executive of the NHS, Nigel Crisp, said: 'Networks R Us'. An editorial in the *British Medical Journal* by the Policy Director of the NHS Confederation, Nigel Edwards, applauded these sentiments (Edwards 2001). However, Edwards drew attention to a series of challenges in networks, including the risk that they might be seen as 'the next structural panacea' and turn into new, centralised NHS organisations. This book hopefully provides a series of reasons why they should not. The fledgling NHS health networks are creatures of the current century. They will need all the help they can get.

## References

Edwards N (2002). Clinical networks. *British Medical Journal* **324**, 63
NHS Eastern Regional Office (2001). Proceedings of a conference: Acute Futures: Organising in a Connected World. NHS Executive, Eastern Region. HMSO

*Roger James* MRCP FRCR
*Andrew Miles* MSc MPhil PhD

## Acknowledgements

We gratefully acknowledge a grant of educational sponsorship from Macmillan Cancer Relief, AstraZeneca UK Ltd and Pfizer Ltd in support of this publication and an associated national conference held at The Royal College of Physicians of London.

Chapter 1

# Managed networks within cancer services: an organisational perspective

*Ewan Ferlie, Chris Hawkins and Beth Kewell*

## Introduction

### Policy background

The 'managed-care network' is a novel mode of organisation and management that is currently being used within the reorganisation of NHS cancer services. It builds on the recommendations of the Calman–Hine Report (1995) which first proposed a networked approach as opposed to a highly centralised approach or a market-led approach. The Calman–Hine Report suggested that cancer centres, units and primary care teams should work in partnership with each other in a network form, with patients being treated at the most appropriate level. Care pathways between the various providers need to be smooth for this model to work. The Calman–Hine Report (1995) also suggested important leadership roles for lead clinician and lead nurses within the implementation process and this may have had the effect of consolidating professional ownership of the model. Network-based working is in any case consistent with the ways in which many healthcare professionals work, albeit this has historically been on a more informal basis and usually only within their own profession.

The network model was a radical proposal at the time – given the then dominant model of the internal market – but has been increasingly accepted by policy-makers. After the change of political control in 1997, overall health policy accorded less stress to the previous guiding ideas of competition and choice and more stress to alternative values: ensuring high quality, and coordinated and integrated care across the whole of the NHS. The policy stress on network-based forms of management within cancer services is strengthening and likely to continue as a major theme over the next 5 years. It is seen as especially appropriate because the 'care pathways' of many cancer patients are complex, likely to cross conventional primary, secondary and tertiary healthcare boundaries, and may also involve social care and some voluntary agencies (such as hospices). Such care pathways can best be managed through a network approach. If successful, this model of the 'managed network' may be exported to other healthcare services, so this is potentially a management innovation of some significance. Note, however, the term 'managed network' implies that it may take a very different form from the tacit and self-regulated professional networks of the past.

## Network building

> There is nothing so practical as a good theory.

> Kurt Lewin

Why do we analyse this development in organisational terms? Many healthcare workers will be primarily interested in their clinical work and see such analysis as of marginal importance. However, the question of whether such managed networks can promote the smoothly flowing care pathways hoped for has enormous practical implications for clinical practitioners. This is an important managerial experiment that needs to be evaluated. A first step within such evaluation is to conceptualise the development: what does theory tell us about managed networks, about the circumstances in which they might and might not be effective?

'Reflective practitioners' (Argyris & Schon 1978) may find that their ability to reflect and conceptualise a complex practical problem helps them frame action strategies. This is particularly the case when organisational models are moving from a received paradigm to a novel paradigm about which there is little practical experience. Many of the key network building roles will be undertaken not only by general managers but by clinical–managerial hybrids (such as clinical directors or 'lead clinicians'). These network builders may find a theoretical base helpful, because they may well be operating across a whole local system and face a complex interorganisational set. They may find organisational diagnostic skills (in addition to their usual clinical diagnostic skills) to be helpful to them in spotting likely areas of forward movement and change resistance. They are now undertaking strategic management roles and may need to develop an additional knowledge base in this field to complement their clinical perspectives.

This chapter seeks to conceptualise the network-based mode of organisation, reviewing some good quality recent studies from inside and outside health care. Second, it outlines some very early empirical results from a management research project that the authors have been conducting which investigates the implementation of the Calman–Hine Report within cancer services. It will conclude with a set of key questions for reflective practitioners.

The literature review includes both generic work and work that has been done specifically in healthcare settings. It is acknowledged that there is no simple 'read across' from private sector to healthcare settings and that this concept may need to be modified to fit NHS work settings. The settings are presented as a preliminary device for expanding 'thought sets' within healthcare management and as an aid to concept building.

## Networks within organisational analysis

At a highly general level, hierarchies, markets and networks have been described as three basic modes of organising (Thompson *et al.* 1991). The mode of co-ordination is through the *command* within hierarchies, through the *price* within markets, and through the *relationship* within networks. The three modes also call for distinctive managerial styles. Thus managers in more market-oriented organisations may take on the persona of an *entrepreneur*, managers in a vertically line-managed organisation take on the persona of *military personnel*, whereas managers in a network-based organisation may take on the persona of a *diplomat*.

The question arises whether there is now a deep-seated shift under way from organisational forms based on markets and hierarchies to a network-based form of organising (the so-called N form) (Nohria & Eccles 1992; Ferlie & Pettigrew 1996; Pettigrew & Fenton 2000). One view is that the last century can be seen as a period dominated by large and 'vertically integrated' (i.e. line-managed) organisations which essentially produced a limited range of standard and mass volume products. Within the private sector, the Ford corporation is an exemplar (this organisational form indeed is often termed 'Fordism'). By the 1980s, these very large corporations were in retreat, as they 'downsized' in order to become more nimble and flexible. Peripheral functions were contracted out or externalised. We used to think that firms would replace markets; now we think that markets replace firms.

Within the public sector, the large Welfare State agencies (such as the NHS) created in the 1940s can be seen as an analogue of the Fordist corporation. However, Fordist models have retained greater resilience in this sector. Vertical integration, if anything, increased in the NHS in the 1980s, with the introduction of general management and the bringing in of the regional offices into the Civil Service. For the first time there was a chain of command (at least in formal terms) throughout the NHS, with a strong performance management orientation, although this coexisted with strong informal professional power.

Since the 1970s, increasing evidence has been accumulating of a very general shift towards more flexible 'post-Fordist' and network-based styles of organising within the private sector. There has been a growth of co-located small entrepreneurial firms, of so-called industrial districts, and of new high-tech sectors that relate to each other on a network basis. Silicon Valley would be an outstanding example of this trend. The following factors are seen as key drivers for the adoption of the N form:

- *Increased requirement for flexibility and learning:* where products are specialised and designed for 'niche markets'; where there is greater service variety and where there is a faster rate of innovation and shorter product cycles; and where there is a need for accelerated organisational as well as individual learning.
- *Requirement to reduce market uncertainty:* stable long-term relationships between suppliers and customers (rather than the use of 'spot transactions') may help provide tacit knowledge about intangible factors such as levels of service and reliability, and hence reduce the level of uncertainty within the market. Much of this tacit knowledge can only be built up slowly through repeated transactions that

slowly build up trust levels. Moreover, the participants need knowledge about others' resources, organisation and development possibilities in order to assess possible future developments. This may lead to a highly 'relational' mode of contracting where long-term relationships of trust emerge between different firms. Indeed, the relationship may become more important than the contract.

- *Need to manage joint production:* there is a move away from sole production to a new form of value-adding partnership (VAP), where a set of independent companies work closely together to manage a flow of goods and services along an entire so-called value-added chain. Low-cost computing and communications systems favour the development of such partnerships of smaller companies, each of which performs one function within the value chain and co-ordinates its activities with the rest. Within the public sector, there are an increasing number of 'joint production' processes involving various components of the NHS, social care and the voluntary sector.

- *A high-tech base:* the shift to the N form is seen as especially strong in high-tech sectors (such as software and biotechnology). These organisations are anchored in knowledge-based industries, where typically there is an alliance between science-based 'start ups' and venture capital. The 'start ups' are small, flexible and located near to other start ups within an industrial district. They typically employ educated, young and mobile professionals with high career expectations. They seek to create new waves of innovative products and must manage novelty and continuous change. The science base is rapidly evolving and implies frequent product redesign.

It would be interesting to plot NHS cancer services against these four dimensions to see how many of these drivers are present.

## Some recent studies of network-based management

NHS organisations have traditionally operated as large-scale, vertically integrated bureaucracies, albeit ones in which professional groups (particularly clinicians) have retained high levels of informal power. The legislatively driven creation of the internal market (1991–97) marked a move to market-based principles of organising, although over time the 'managed market' became more managed and less of a market (Mays *et al.* 2000). Some healthcare services (community health services, mental health) have long operated in a network-based fashion, although in a more tacit and 'unmanaged' way. By the mid-1990s, there was some evidence that other healthcare organisations were attempting to move to a more network-based mode of organising.

### Ferlie and Pettigrew (1996)

This article explored whether the new purchasing organisations set up in 1991 were moving towards more of a network form than the old district health authorities

(DHAs). It was apparent that much of the purchasing agenda revolved around the construction of interagency alliances where traditional notions of 'command and control' were inappropriate. Alliances with local government, community organisations and economic agencies were being developed at a strategic level. Internally, there were reports of moves to matrix-based and more fluid structures within the new purchasing organisations. A key role of the chief executive officer (CEO) was to undertake the 'foreign policy' component of the agenda, with the delegation of the internal operational agenda. The winning of influence was, in these circumstances, more important that the direct exercise of power.

The study concluded that network-based styles of management were indeed of substantial and rising importance, but that this marked a shift of emphasis rather than total displacement of one mode by another. Respondents talked of the need to operate in different modes in different circumstances, and CEOs still needed to ensure performance management. They also needed to 'meta-manage' the many networks that had emerged, putting effort into promising sectors and perhaps withdrawing from those that were not purposeful enough.

When asked to define the characteristics and skills needed within network-based forms of management, words such as 'trust', 'reciprocity', 'understanding' and 'credibility' all emerged as basic concepts in use. There is thus an important interpersonal component to network-based forms of management, which can make it vulnerable to turnover of key people. However, the alignment of incentives at an agency level is also important because it is unlikely that decision-makers from different agencies will work together unless a 'win–win' situation is constructed. As coercive or manipulative forms of behaviour are unlikely to be successful, achieving such interorganisational trust may be considerably more difficult than building interpersonal networks, yet vital if alliances are to survive the departure of key individuals.

Criticisms of network-based approaches included:

- They were very time-consuming and the relationship to organisational performance was not always clear; there could be a rapid proliferation of different networks.
- It was difficult to sustain these networks in the long run, particularly if they did not deliver early output valued by all parties; participants might well decide to withdraw from non-productive networks.
- Network building is a slow, emergent and long-term process, conflicting with short-term and task-led approaches to performance management. This is particularly the case if non-governmental actors (community-based or voluntary organisations) are included; indeed government can here lose direct control with a move to a shared power model.
- Networks could promote conservatism as well as change, excluding new actors and new ideas; they could become very closed systems with a small number of highly embedded players.

- The HRM implications and issues of the move to network-based working had not been thought through fully, although there was a requirement for different managerial styles and knowledge bases.

This early study was important because it was one of the first to spot the empirical growth of network-based approaches within the NHS and tried to conceptualise them.

## Dennison (1997): a process model of organisations

In the NHS, as elsewhere, a suite of so-called change initiatives was introduced throughout the 1990s (total quality management [TQM]; business process re-engineering; breakthrough collaboratives; network-based organisations; process redesign; care pathways). Although often analysed singly, they can also be seen as a family of interventions, all of which attempt to shift healthcare services from a traditional vertical pattern of organising to a novel lateral model of organising.

At this higher level, Dennison (1997) has described a so-called 'process model' of organisations in which contemporary firms are being organised in terms of their underlying 'value chain'. A value chain (Porter 1985) is conceived of as a linked system of independent activities that are the building blocks of a firm's competitive advantage, such as the chain made up of research and design (R&D), engineering, manufacturing, and sales and marketing activities.

Organisations are seen in this model as a collection of processes that add value for the customer. Such value creation is a non-hierarchical process that involves the lateral co-ordination of a chain of events taking place inside and outside the boundaries of a formal organisation in response to market-based feedback. The 'job' of an organisation is to define the optimal value chain and then to establish appropriate relationships between the steps. The most important source of guidance is not control by hierarchy but external control by customers, through feedback and input.

Within more 'virtually based' organisations, there may be a system of individual organisations – large and small – which focus on one segment of the distribution chain, while relying on outsourced supply and distribution partners up- and downstream to provide other links in the value chain. These relationships are market based and governed by contracts as well as interpersonal relations of trust. Such process-based organisations certainly do not exhibit layers of hierarchy, long chains of command, complex decision-making processes and highly developed bureaucracies. The notion of a 'value chain' is highly linear and mechanistic; that of a 'value network' is more organic, allowing for interaction and feedback loops.

The analogy with re-engineering, process redesign and the care pathways models being increasingly used within healthcare services is clearly evident. One problem is that these lateral modes of organisation remain weak in terms of resources and governance structures, coexisting with traditional vertical lines (e.g. trusts, clinical directorates and specialities) which remain resilient and which may impede care transitions across organisational boundaries. A second problem is that the range of professional groupings also evident within healthcare organisations have historically acted to protect and enhance their 'jurisdictions' (Abbott 1988) and blocked radical moves to role blurring and multidisciplinarity.

## Pettigrew and Fenton (2000)

Pettigrew and Fenton's important recent study (2000) explored the extent to which there had been a shift to the N form of organising in a sample of European private sector firms, using both surveys and case studies. They argued that change to a network form could be assessed through movement along three different dimensions:

- structure
- processes and
- boundaries

and they developed subindicators within each of these core dimensions to assess the extent of change, e.g. they found substantial increases in the degree of horizontal interactions reported in the study period (1992–96) such as the greater sharing of R&D knowledge across units and joint purchasing. However, the development of new information technology (IT) and human resouce management systems were needed to underpin these new ways of lateral working. The shift to the N form was still partial and could proceed over a long time frame.

They then explored the relationship between the extent and type of change reported and data on firm performance. They found that higher levels of performance were associated with system-wide change (i.e. to structure, process and boundaries) and that partial change could in fact have negative performance consequences. However, even in the high change firms, there was still a role for the hierarchy as well as the network. There was a series of dualities to be managed including:

- greater performance accountability upwards and horizontal integration sideways
- empowering and holding the ring
- centralising strategy and decentralising operations.

Possible learning points from this study for the NHS include:

- the danger of relying on purely structural forms of change
- the need to develop IT and HRM systems which reinforce moves to network-based working
- that any shift to network-based forms of working may proceed over a long time frame as skills and learning capacity build up slowly

- that performance levels may increase only where there is system-wide change towards network-based working
- a change in the role of the centre towards framework setting and 'holding the ring' rather than operational management.

## Networks in cancer services – some early empirical evidence

In this section, some early empirical evidence generated by our research project on changes to the organisation and management of cancer services is reported.

### Regional implementation style

Stage 1 of the project consisted of an initial round of interviews with regional office (RO) personnel. The RO interviews (Kewell *et al.* 2000a) suggested that substantial variation in regional strategies could be discerned, at least in the early stages of the implementation of the Calman–Hine Report, sometimes reflecting the overall management style of the region. After 1997, there were attempts to move to a more consistent style of implementation across the regions. All regions attempted to support the establishment of cancer networks and some form of accreditation mechanism.

Regions drove the designation and accreditation process for cancer centres and units. One grouping of 'hands-on' regions espoused a planned strategic change approach which equated closely with a purchaser (now commissioner)-led model of service change. Here RO staff perceived themselves as 'market umpires' and then as active performance managers, setting milestones for accreditation in a way that replicated regional performance management systems. Although there was a high pace of top-down change and short-term performance targets were met, the danger that these regions faced was losing the benefit of bottom-up support from DHAs, providers and practitioners. Nursing staff and professions allied to medicine (PAM) were not always fully included in the decision-making machinery. In one region, the Calman–Hine Report was used as a top-down driver organised around a patient pathway approach, but in a way that was challenging to existing clinical practices.

In a second group of 'light touch' regions, staff presented themselves as being more affirmatively led by clinical professional rationales and patient needs. Emergent networks were crafted around ad-hoc and informal professional allegiances and were inclusive of the nursing and PAM professions. These consensual approaches built up long-term trust, but were also subject to delays and bottlenecks which could threaten the pace of change. The danger here is also that very poor clinical practice is not exposed early enough. However, such networks are more likely to generate long-term commitment from clinical professionals.

A subset of regions tried to balance performance management and bottom-up ownership and this is potentially a powerful combination for change, if it can be sustained. Clearly, the nature of the regional implementation strategy was one important factor that could shape the emergence of networks at local level.

## Local centres and networks – structure

The RO interviews were followed up by a postal questionnaire which went to the 36 lead clinicians of cancer centres (30) and networks (6) that we were able to identify nationally. The questions asked were mainly of a structural nature, making the questionnaire easier to fill in for respondents. Twenty were returned, giving a satisfactory response rate of 56%.

### Low and high complexity

The questionnaire data suggested (Kewell *et al*. 2000b) two distinct groupings of networks. Group A consisted of smaller centres, with the number of units reported ranging only from one to two. In the larger group B centres, by contrast, the number of units reported ranged from 1 up to 19. The high level of network complexity in the larger group poses particular management challenges. The number of smaller centres is perhaps greater than envisaged in the Calman–Hine Report.

### Network type

Of 20 centres, 19 indicated that they were affiliated to a cancer care network but we could distinguish two contrasting types of centre unit collaboration. What we might describe as *level 1* collaboration involves extending the work performed by multidisciplinary teams (MDTs) (based at centres) to include outreach to units (18 of 20 responses indicated that there was consultant outreach to units; 16 of 19 responses indicated that there were common treatment and referral protocols). It can be seen as more of a 'hub-and-spoke approach' than a true network. It is essentially unidirectional outreach from centres to units.

*Level 2* collaboration incorporates level 1 activity but goes beyond it to include more education and training activity, and hence provide an environment of shared organisational learning involving: continuous professional development (CPD), shared workforce planning, and joint training and staff rotation plans. We suggest that this model is better able to respond to the Calman–Hine vision of an N form than the more restricted 'hub-and-spoke' model apparent within type 1. Based on answers to type 2 indicators, our estimate is that about 40% of centres were at the time of the survey at level 1, whereas about 60% had moved on to level 2.

### Single and multiple centres

The survey also found that about 50% of centres were based within a single acute trust, but not necessarily on just one hospital site. These *single centres* faced a simpler organisational situation than *multiple centres* (again about 50%) which could straddle two or even more acute trusts, and perhaps also a community trust. Within these multiple centres, there were complex issues of strategic management which would re-emerge when proposals for service rationalisation were made.

## Leadership

Organisational leadership in the network was another theme. Most networks reported that clinicians had been appointed to lead clinician role within the component sites. However, the network as a whole was more frequently chaired by a trust CEO or a senior DHA member. The division of leadership roles between clinicians and senior lay managers remains an interesting question, but the former appear to have retained important formal roles.

## Local centres and networks – process

Stage 2 of our study consists of a set of eight local case studies (one in each region, stratified sample selected on the size dimension) and is still ongoing. Here we report very early details from five sites where empirical work has been undertaken. The case study module can provide evidence of organisational process to complement the structural data gained through the survey.

All the five sites visited so far have moved from the initial designation and accreditation processes to a *gradual formalisation of networks*. This is perceived by clinicians as a positive move from the old centre/unit debate that created conflict. That conflict was often centred on perceptions of differential status and power, and the levels of resources that went with them. It was perceived by management and clinicians that being a designated cancer unit carried less status than being a centre. It was also believed that less money would be available for service development within units. Trusts that had existing good external relationships and were used to working together had fewer problems with these issues and were able to develop their services in a more coherent way from the outset.

### Trust mergers

Where trust mergers were either taking place or being negotiated, the development of cancer networks has often been delayed. One might have thought that mergers would be an ideal opportunity to re-evaluate and reorganise services. It may be that concentration on organisational issues rather than disease specific activity has resulted in struggles to retain strategic control between those organisations undergoing mergers and that this has led to 'planning blight'. This suggests that there may be low levels of trust within some networks, with power struggles and 'gaming' to retain a service presence.

### Flawed local histories

There are bad as well as good local histories which operate at three different levels: the interpersonal, interprofessional and interorganisational levels. The inheritance from the past plays a large role in shaping the pace of service development. More positively, there seems to be a general move from a uniprofessional (medically dominated) to a more multiprofessional system with the creation of MDTs. Most see this as a legitimate challenge and are very positive about improving services through working in a more multidisciplinary way which may act to improve the tenor of interpersonal and interprofessional relations.

Changes in the organisation of *primary care* have to date limited the participation of GPs in the formation of cancer services, but networks are now trying to increase primary care representation.

## Network formalisation and its limits

There is local variation but the overall trend is towards network formalisation. The managers of these formalised networks are not yet decided in all instances. In some places, the management team appears to be similar in structure to that of a trust, with representation from all participating organisations. They will form a network management board under which various groups will be formed to deal with strategic issues.

At the level of clinical practice, there is a growth in the production of protocols, guidelines and care pathways which again represents a formalisation of practice at that level. This has been reinforced by the development of national level standards.

However, resource allocation continues to be dealt with by the individual trusts. There appears (as yet) to be no plan to allow the network to hold its own resource base. Discussions are taking place about the commissioning role of the health authorities (HAs) and primary care teams (PCTs), and how the changed structure might affect the resourcing of the cancer networks. Governance arrangements are formally still through lines of accountability to trusts and HAs, mixed with self-regulation through professional bodies.

## Some questions arising

Combining our original theoretical review with some early empirical data, some wider questions emerge.

### Can one combine network-based management and performance management?

This appears pragmatically to be happening at the moment. Critics argue that there is a possibility of a contradiction between the two because networks cannot be externally performance managed in a manner that would be usual in a command and control organisation. To what extent can the chair of a network be expected to control the behaviour of other network members who may be from different healthcare organisations or from outside the NHS altogether? Yet it is the network chair who is likely to be held accountable for network development through the performance management line.

British public sector management is strongly dominated by narrow notions of performance management when viewed in an international perspective, e.g. the account of policy networks of Kickert *et al.* (1997) which are particularly strong within the Dutch public management tradition stresses the emergent, bottom-up and unexpected components of network-based management. Government is only one of many actors and has no power to determine the behaviour of other stakeholders. Network-based management requires a long and exhaustive process of consensus building and problem definition before joint action can be taken and any change can be made to 'stick.'

Some would say that this tension is a paradox rather than a contradiction. There is some evidence that successful managers are those who have a repertoire of approaches, and who can switch styles according to the problem in hand (O'Neill & Quinn 1993). Internal performance management of the network by its own members would be an alternative solution.

### What are the governance and accountability arrangements for networks?

Is the new lateral organisation to remain no more than a weak layer laid across the traditional vertical forms which in the end reassert their dominance? This depends in part on whether professional groups seek narrowly to defend their jurisdictions or whether they are willing to share tasks with other professions in a broader way. It also depends on where budgetary and strategic authority lie. This raises the question of governance and accountability arrangements for these new networks, as well as their degree of control over resource flows.

There is a further question about who is in the network. In particular, will it be restricted to a tertiary to secondary care network, or will it also include primary care (which appears to be weakly represented at the moment), social care and the voluntary sector? If the latter agencies come in, then it will be even more difficult to operate in an externally driven performance management style, because they remain outside the NHS.

## Distribution of power and influence within the network

We believe that the underlying distribution of power and influence within a network is an important consideration. Power imbalance may pave the way to an attempt to dominate by the most powerful partner and withdrawal from the network by the less powerful. So the operation of networks may be constrained when there is an overt contest for power and influence between their various stakeholders. It is of course possible to construct 'win–win' situations which avoid such power struggle. There is evidence of a gradual loosening of medical dominance and a move to more multidisciplinary working, yet this is welcomed by many clinicians themselves as an improved form of service delivery. Yet interorganisational power conflicts, e.g. over proposed mergers or service rationalisations, are certainly apparent and may prevent network development at a more strategic level.

## Too much non-reflective practice

We believe the management challenges in N form organisations to be distinctive and to be worthy of reflection. We have found that frontline managers are so immersed in a busy operational change agenda that they are often unable to consider these issues, or to talk about how network management is different from command and control management. Network management may be easier for doctors to understand (because they have always operated within the context of strong professional networks) than managers or indeed nurses who are used to working within a hierarchy.

Yet, as networks consolidate, so there will be important changes in the roles undertaken by managers in cancer services. As Pettigrew and Fenton argue, such as shift needs to be supported by HRM systems (and we would add the education and training and also the R&D systems) if it is to have positive effects. At the moment, there is in our view a need to develop a culture of reflective managerial practice in order to explore these issues further.

## Acknowledgements

We are grateful to NHS London R&D (O and M Group) for funding the empirical study on which this paper draws.

## *References*

Abbott A (1988). *The System of Professions*. London: University of Chicago Press

Argyris C & Schon E (1978). *Organisational Learning*. Reading, MA: Addison Wesley

Calman–Hine Report (1995). *A Policy Framework for Commissioning Cancer Services*. London: Department of Health

Denison DR (1977). Towards a process based theory of organisational designs. *Advances in Strategic Management* **14**, 1–44

Ferlie E & Pettigrew A (1996). Managing through networks: some issues and implications for the NHS. *British Journal of Management* **7**, S81–S99

Kewell B, Ferlie E, Hawkins C (2000a). *From Market Umpires to Relationship Managers? The Future of NHS ROs in a Time of Transition*. Bristol: Bristol Business School

Kewell B, Ferlie E, Hawkins C (2000b). *Assessing The Legacy of Calman Hine: A Study of Organisational Change Amongst Cancer Services in England*. Bristol: Business School

Kickert W, Klijn E, Koppenjan J (1997). *Managing Complex Networks*. London: Sage

Mays N, Mulligan JA, Goodwin N (2000). The British quasi market in healthcare: a review of the evidence. *Journal of Health Services Research and Policy* **5**, 49–58

Nohria N & Eccles R (eds) (1992). *Networks and Organizations: Structure, form and action*. Cambridge, MA: Harvard Business School Press

O'Neill R & Quinn RE (1993). Applications of the competing values framework. *Human Resource Management* **32**, 1–7

Pettigrew A & Fenton E (2000). *The Innovating Organisation*. London: Sage

Porter M (1985). *Competitive Advantage*. New York: Free Press

Thompson G, Frances J, Levacic R, Mitchell J (1991). *Markets, Hierarchies and Networks*. London: Sage

# Chapter 2

# Definitions of care networks within the National Health Service

*Peter Spurgeon and Liz Watson*

## Introduction

Since the advent of a new UK government in 1997 there has been a rejection of the previous experiment with the internal market in health care. This has been replaced by an emphasis, in terms of both explicit policy statements and practice, on collaboration between health organisations. The Cancer Collaborative is an example of a disease-based collaboration whereas the hub-and-spoke model illustrates typically large and small organisations joining together to offer services in a different way. A number of pressures have combined to direct health care in this particular way and these forces are discussed later.

The concept of network might well be the best single collective term to describe these collaborative approaches. However, it is clear that a number of different terms have emerged over the past two decades (e.g. care pathways, integrated care, managed care and clinical networks), all relating to the notion of managed care, whether within or between institutions. Inevitably, as time and practice evolve, there is slippage in meaning and a degree of overlap in what exactly is meant by each specific label. It may be useful therefore to attempt to provide a definition, and more importantly an implication, of each term.

## Definitions and implications

Managed care is perhaps the earliest form, at least in the USA, although it is subsequently to be found in the UK attached to integrated care pathways and collaborative care programmes (Ellis 1997). Managed care covers a spectrum of activities carried out in various organisational settings. It is argued by Fairfield *et al.* (1997) that whatever the activities the common aim is to modify professional behaviour towards cost-effective care.

In the USA, managed care came to the fore in the 1980s when it was directed particularly to containing spiralling healthcare costs. Indeed it is suggested that the managed-care process did succeed in reducing costs by between 6 and 7% (Gottlieb 1996). The insurance-based financing of health care in the USA inevitably meant that managed care was focused on the hypothetical patient and condition, allowing an estimate of what sort of cost might be expected from a specified set of treatments and procedures. Although managed-care programmes appeared to obtain a degree of success in controlling costs, the process appeared to give less emphasis to improvements in quality. For this reason the approach was viewed with some scepticism and therefore resistance by clinicians, particularly in the UK. It was regarded as imposing excessive documentation and challenging the appropriateness of certain treatments. Early UK initiatives were hampered by this perspective.

However, the concept has evolved and in the UK the term 'managed care' has incorporated collaborative care programming and care pathways. Although this multiple terminology may add to confusion, the importance of the UK-based development of the concept is that it has given a counterbalancing greater emphasis to quality and consistency of care. The latter of course resonates firmly with the government's current concern to eliminate inconsistent standards of care. Care pathways represent a systems approach that concentrates on a specific disease or condition and the management of it. The care pathway describes the relevant clinical care, the chronology of this treatment and in many cases the expected outcome.

De Luc and Currie (1999) reviewed the origin and purpose of many care pathway developments. They suggest most had as their objective one or more of the following:

- controlling or minimising costs of improving resource utilisation
- co-ordinating care to produce greater consistency and to avoid duplication
- improving patient documentation
- supporting evidence-based practice and the implementation of clinical guidelines
- enhancing the cycle of clinical audit through the analysis of variations from the pathway
- supporting the provision of seamless care by developing pathways across health (and social care) sectors
- providing a currency for future contracting or commissioning
- allowing for benchmarking of performance both within and across organisations.

The new philosophy of health care as evidenced in the government's White Paper *The New NHS: Modern dependable* gave further impetus to the use of care pathways (Department of Health 1997). The increasingly multidisciplinary nature of pathways linked helpfully to allow changes within the health system, which highlighted the need for more teamwork in the delivery of care involving a range of professionals. The drive towards evidence-based medicine was also felt to be supported by the use of pathways as a means of ensuring more consistency in the care process. Finally, the strengthening of primary care and specifically primary care trusts has reinforced the need to develop pathways that promote seamless care across the health sectors.

There are of course a host of difficulties in the successful implementation of the ideal concept of care pathways. However, the third form of network is perhaps the most radical and challenging, the managed clinical network. The concept was clearly defined by the Scottish Department of Health in 1999, following a review of acute services in Scotland, in a Management Executive Letter (1999). The document defined managed clinical networks as 'linked groups of health professionals and organisations from primary, secondary and tertiary care, working in a co-ordinated manner, unconstrained by existing professional and health board boundaries, to ensure equitable provision of high quality, clinically effective services throughout Scotland'.

A similar conception has been propounded by the Health Department of Western Australia within their plan for health care in the twenty-first century. Using a slightly different name, they describe integrated clinical services as 'promoting the seamless movement of health professionals and patient care across hospital and health service boundaries so that health services can operate as one metropolitan-wide service incorporating promotion and prevention, diagnostic and acute care and continuing care services'.

The common and most radical idea within both definitions is the notion that health professionals, including doctors, will work within a service framework that is determined by patient need and by the nature of the provision, but no longer constrained by institutional boundaries. Traditionally, the organisation and management of health services has been subsumed by the hospital or health services in which they operate. Clinicians have, in the main, operated within the boundaries of the services delivered by particular hospitals, with occasional outreach services.

The development of managed clinical network for cardiology in Scotland is described by Baker and Lorimer (2000). It can be seen that many of the expected components of care pathways are contained within their description. Managed clinical networks are suggested as promoting greater consistency of practice, facilitating local provision and thereby better access, as well as improving co-ordination between sectors. In addition, the network is seen as the focus of teaching and education and research, and ultimately new forms of resource allocation outside existing individual institutions.

## Forces leading towards network-based services

McKee *et al.* (1998) suggest that there have been parallel processes of organisational change in health organisations which have reinforced these developments. Hospitals in particular have been exhorted to increase their efficiency and yet, at the same time, there has been a demand to improve access and to provide services as close to people's homes as possible. There are obvious tensions here and in some ways networks represent an attempt to offer a compromise. A number of the forces to change are common to health systems across the world.

The position of the hospital as the central organisation is undoubtedly in a state of flux. In the USA, many hospitals have closed and the relationship between the hospital and the community it serves is being re-negotiated. In most European health systems, the number of hospital beds has reduced significantly over the past decade.

The situation is, however, complex with some of the processes of particularly high technology-based medicine driving towards a centralisation on to large hospital sites, while at the same time electronic information transfer makes it possible to deliver services even closer to the patient's home.

Clark *et al.* (2000) examined the key forces for health reform affecting systems across the world. Some of the key factors identified are presented in Table 2.1.

**Table 2.1** Driving forces for change

Demographic shifts in the population creating a tension between physical location of hospital systems and the community need

An emphasis on developing primary and community-based care as an alternative to hospital-based provision

The demands of medical education and training requiring collaboration between hospitals so as to ensure an appropriate educative experience

A demand for greater equality of access and consistency of treatments and outcomes between different hospitals

Changes in clinical practice, in part based on new technology, but also an increased degree of subspecialisation again necessitating greater inter-organisational collaboration

A need to recognise the demands of the clinical governance agenda and risk management with particular reference to providing the appropriate level of medical cover (especially in the context of emergency work)

From Clark *et al.* (2000).

The physical geography, financing framework and social conditions existing within individual health systems obviously exert some influence on how the impact of the above forces is resolved.

## The challenge of networks

The flexibility and diffuse nature of the network concept require a very clear structure of roles and accountability within it because the old institutional hierarchies will no longer function. There is a vital need for a high level of involvement and leadership from clinicians, but at the same time this key group is feeling destabilised by the disappearing identity and loyalty to a familiar institutional base. Identification with a virtual network is obviously difficult to foster and will require a major change in attitude.

The shift in focus of patient activity to the network framework also poses major question marks over the financial and contracting processes. The traditional allocation of resources in budget envelopes to institutions is convenient and tidy. However, if the reality is that patients will move across institutions within a clinical network, there will need to be some parallel flow of resources to match the new pattern.

The key requirements of a network will be the appropriate provision of the facilities and infrastructure to deliver the care as and where required in a place convenient to the patient. This, in turn, will place a renewed focus on efficient facilities management at various sites within the network. Again this will require a change in the nature of the management task.

Although networks, similar to care pathways, are a natural focus for evidence-based medicine, they will also need to develop mechanisms for dealing with the increasing co-morbidity of patients, which might in principle challenge the boundaries of the network.

In the next section we look at how the establishment of a new network has been tackled in a specific example location.

## Planning emerging clinical networks in a health economy

Plans to 'modernise' the health economies will, in general, require a complete re-design of services from a whole-system perspective. The success of these plans will involve the removal of institutional barriers, and the emergence of networks of clinical and social care professionals working in hospital and community settings. Clinicians will work together across organisational boundaries and locations of care.

In the future, patients with a chronic and/or acute clinical condition may receive care from a care team which may consist of many health and social care professionals. Where patients have complex needs, their care may need to be co-ordinated across speciality-based teams. Professionals in the care team may have dual accountability: on a discipline basis and as a member of a multidisciplinary team whose members work together to manage an individual's healthcare needs. A clinician may be a member of one or more clinical teams, depending on the needs of the individual patient.

### Planning assumptions

The concept of a managed clinical network assumes that benefits can be obtained in the quality of care provided to individuals by clinicians in a team providing care across different physical locations. In developing the management options for clinical networks, a number of assumptions emerge which need to be critically appraised.

It is assumed, for example, that an unambiguous and consistent process of care can be described for individual patients and populations. This process of care may indicate, at a very detailed level, the expected clinical decisions required for the use of health resources given certain clinical indications, e.g. when certain diagnostic tests should be used. The process of care may also refer to the patient pathway through different locations of care and teams: a less detailed investigation of the care pathway. The two planning activities have different purposes: the former to assist clinicians in detailed clinical decision-making, the latter to answer planning questions such as the number and location of intermediate care beds.

If clinical teams work across multiple locations, it is assumed that the right level of supervision can be provided to ensure clinical safety. This supervision may require changes to existing clinical practice through, for example, greater use of clinical protocols or accreditation for provision of certain types of service.

Reorienting the focus of the clinical team away from the organisation, giving the team flexibility in the way in which different locations of care can be used, means that patient-based, clinical information must be accessible by professionals wherever a patient consultation occurs. It also requires the members of clinical teams to share information about the care that has been provided in a meaningful away across multiple disciplines. An efficient clinical network therefore also requires detailed clinical information to be available in real time, i.e. there should be no time lag between the availability of the information and its collection. Professionals will need to record information during a consultation.

The implementation of clinical networks enables a separation between the management of facilities and the management of clinical teams. If the holistic needs of the patient are considered and if the care that an individual receives can be provided in many possible locations, a team may no longer be defined by the facility in which it works. There is therefore an opportunity to separate out the management of facilities from the management of clinical networks.

A clinical network may also offer the opportunity to redefine organisational boundaries on the basis of the management of facilities and management of clinical teams. However, the impact of organisational reconfigurations on the effectiveness of clinical teams is unclear.

In some cases, a professional group may still be bound by a facility because of the nature of their work. In such cases the implementation of clinical networks in other areas that consist of logical groups of specialities or targeted at population groups may create new boundaries to the efficient delivery of care. Similarly, if the use of step-down facilities in community settings for population groups such as frail elderly people are not supported by a strong ethos of rehabilitation, existing bottlenecks in the use of health resources may be recreated elsewhere. The effectiveness of the network may therefore be diluted unless there is a whole-system change to the way in which care is delivered.

The successful implementation of clinical networks that achieve expected improvements in efficiency and clinical effectiveness will rely on the following:

- Implementation of clear patient management processes within and across clinical teams within a framework for clinical accountability.
- Sophisticated use of information and technology to ensure timely access to information.

- Significant cultural change among professional groups to develop clinical teams centred around the needs of the individual patient.

None of these is necessarily dependent on the implementation of clinical networks, but should be features of all 'modern' health services. The lack of sufficient information technology support systems, for example, has been shown to be a limiting factor in developing care plans as working documents (Silagy *et al.* 1999).

## Management options

Working from the multiple definitions to date, there are three broad management options for the development of clinical networks. These are:

- facility to facility
- speciality based
- co-ordinator.

### Facility to facility

The current situation can be broadly described as separate clinical teams working mainly within facilities. For clinical networks to be implemented, protocols for the transfer of care from one clinical team to another and a consistent approach to care management need to be agreed. There would be minimal change to existing arrangements for the management of clinical teams within organisations, although work on clinical pathways and process changes within facilities would need to be undertaken. Managers of facilities would continue also to manage clinical teams. Commissioning would continue to be undertaken on a facility-by-facility basis within a strategic framework for each patient group.

### Speciality-based model

The model in Figure 2.1 describes how specialists who mainly provide care in secondary and tertiary environments may work together in networks of care. The model already exists in, for example, cancer services. The specialist care network would include outreach services provided, for example, by specialist nurses to patients in their homes. Specialist clinicians would also work closely with other professionals, such as general practitioners, to ensure the implementation of clearly defined care pathways for patients with conditions that can be managed in primary care.

A balance needs to be achieved between the management of a patient's clinical condition and his or her other multiple health and social needs. This model might be too narrow for patients with multiple health and social care needs, and therefore may be applicable only to those patients who need to receive episodic care or for whom most of their needs can be met by a single speciality. These speciality-based networks

**Speciality-based team**

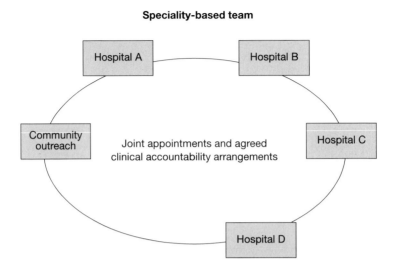

**Figure 2.1** Speciality-based model.

will still require careful management of the interface with other care providers to ensure that the total needs of the patient are met.

In this model the management of facilities can be separated out from the management of clinical teams. Boundaries between clinical teams and between the clinical teams and facilities' managers would need to be carefully managed.

This model would support the implementation of service-based commissioning across speciality-based groups. Where clinical speciality-based networks spanned multiple organisations, lead commissioning arrangements would be possible.

## Co-ordinator model

In the model in Figure 2.2, a member of the primary care team interfaces between multiple health and social care providers and speciality-based networks, integrating care plans and co-ordinating the care required. The total needs of the client are managed by the care co-ordinator who is accountable for ensuring that providers of care work together to meet the needs of the individual. Clinical accountability would depend on the range of the needs of the individual.

This model is most appropriate to those patients with complex health and social care needs requiring care from multidisciplinary teams. Co-ordinated care also offers opportunities to remove administrative barriers to change by enabling, for example, pooled budgets where the co-ordinator of care would be responsible for commissioning care with other providers. There would be an opportunity for the implementation of

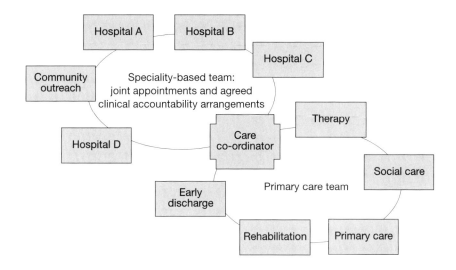

**Figure 2.2** Co-ordinator model.

'managed care' where the co-ordinator of care, as fundholder, would have an incentive to change investment for more appropriate community-based interventions. However, this would need to be balanced by monitoring of access to services to ensure that disincentives were not introduced into the system which could create barriers for access. This model is the most radical departure from current practice.

## Implementation of different models

No one model is clearly better than any other. Each model creates boundaries that will need to be managed. A key theme, even with existing facility-to-facility networks, is the importance of effective protocols for the transfer of a patient's clinical management across boundaries. Whole-system management will require all clinical teams to manage system components, with a view to improving the system performance as a whole. This will be true whichever type of network model is adopted.

The co-ordinator model has the potential to introduce the right incentives into the system because the co-ordinator is responsible for the whole of a person's care needs and can therefore integrate different system components. However, evidence of its effectiveness is lacking at this stage (Silage *et al.* 1999). The co-ordinator of care model does not obviate the need for processes to be agreed between different clinical teams and other components of the system.

Interim results from the co-ordinated care trials in Australia (Silagy *et al.* 1999) have highlighted some of the difficulties in achieving demonstrable improvements to health outcomes. Nine trials have recruited 16,533 clients with complex and chronic health needs, i.e. with an unstable medical condition, low level of social support and/or a severe chronic illness. The evidence to date suggests that there is great variability in co-ordinated care models. Their effect on client health and well-being, service cost and use, hospitalisation, re-admission and length of stay is inconclusive. It is hoped that more conclusive evidence will become available through future evaluation reports at the end of the trial. However, the evaluators make it clear that:

> . . . local ownership of care coordination is important, as long as this does not create
> unnecessary duplication of existing health care management structures; and in order
> to be effective, coordinated care requires a primary care team approach, with GPs
> playing an important and integral part.

Multiple models of clinical networks may coexist depending on the needs of the patient. Successful implementation will require a staged approach to implementation. In the short term, it may be viewed as more urgent to streamline process issues between existing boundaries, in order to change the culture towards more joint working across organisations and interdisciplinary teams. In some communities senior clinicians from primary and secondary care are already leading the development of these pathways.

Re-design of the patient journey requires changes not only to clinical and management practice, but also to the strategy development process. Instead of focusing on the nature and location of facilities, strategies will need to describe the new patient journey through the health and social care system. This new planning process will allow better strategic alignment among health, information management and technology (IM&T), human resource and organisational development strategies. Investment decisions in 'infrastructure' can be explicitly tied to the achievement of health strategy goals.

## Conclusion

Clinical networks intuitively offer the potential for achieving quality improvements to the NHS. However, there are many definitions and a lack of clarity about their scope and purpose. Recent legislative changes such as the Health Act 1999 and policy direction, such as additional investment in IM&T and removal of outmoded professional demarcations, are necessary prerequisites to implementing clinical networks. The greatest challenge will be for local communities to define their own response to broad policy direction: to move beyond a technocratic approach to network definition, towards an organisational culture that achieves improvement in care delivery which is focused on the needs of the patients.

## *References*

Baker CD & Lorimer AR (2000). Cardiology: the development of a managed clinical network. *British Medical Journal* **321**, 1152–1153

Clark J, Skinner C, Spurgeon P (2000). *International Critique of Integrated Clinical Services*. Health Services Management Centre, University of Birmingham de Luc K & Currie L (1999). *Developing, Implementing and Evaluating Care Pathways in the UK: The Way to Go.* Health Services Management Centre Research Report 34, University of Birmingham

Department of Health (1997). *The New NHS: Modern, dependable.* London: HMSO

Ellis BW (1997). Managed care: a hospital clinician's view. *Journal of Managed Care* **1**, 9–11

Fairfield G, Hunter D, Mechanic D, Fleming R (1997). Managed care: origins, principles and evolutions. *British Medical Journal* **314**, 1823–1826

Gottlieb S (1996). The role of managed care in financing medical education: a survey of views. *Journal of the American Medical Association* **276**, 750–762

McKee M, Aiken L, Rafferty AM, Sochalski J (1998) Organisational change and quality of health care: an evolving international agenda. *Quality in Health Care* **7**, 37–41

Management Executive Letter (1999). *The Introduction of Managed Clinical Networks within the NHS in Scotland.* Scottish Office, Department of Health, Edinburgh

Silagy C, Brett F, Leigh J *et al.* (1999). Commonwealth Department of Health and Aged Care, The Australian Coordinated Care Trial. *Interim National Evaluation Summary.* September

Chapter 3

# The role of pharmaceutical companies in managed-care networks

*Beverley Salt*

## Introduction

This chapter provides an insight into the role and development of managed-care organisations (MCOs). It starts with an explanation of what an MCO actually is and then discusses the success of the initiatives to date. The chapter then moves on to an objective analysis of the relationship between MCOs and the pharmaceutical industry. It identifies some of the barriers to be faced with the collaboration process, which will provide challenges for the future. A case-management model of cancer is discussed to highlight the practical implications of managed care. Finally, the chapter points to the positive impact that MCOs and pharmaceutical companies can bring in tandem: by providing more efficient diagnosis and disease management, producing increased survival rates and a higher quality of long-term care.

## What are managed-care networks?

Managed-care networks were first developed in the mid-1980s in the USA as an alternative to the traditional fee-for-service system, in which those who pay for health care exert little influence over its delivery. Managed care provides services to a circumscribed patient population for a monthly capitation payment intended to cover the full array of healthcare services. The growth of managed care has been very rapid in recent years. In 1991, 4.9 million Medicare and Medicaid recipients were being covered in MCOs; this figure increased to 7.1 million in 1993 and 17.6 million in 1995 (Baronas 1995). In 1996, Medicare patients were signing up with MCOs at a rate of 70,000 per month (Muirhead 1996).

Managed care was established as a means of emphasising cost control, access for all and promotion of quality (Ellwood & Lundberg 1996). Under the best circumstances, managed care controls costs and promotes quality of care by reducing inefficient variation in practice (Krumholz 1999). Only 5 years after its establishment, the American health system had run up unanticipated costs, forcing the Department of Health, Education and Welfare to implement reform. The result was a unique American approach combining social insurance with market forces (Ellwood & Lundberg 1996). The new health plans grew in membership in the mid-1980s when, faced with the prospect of intensifying global competition for sale of products and uncontrollable healthcare costs, employer purchasers began seriously encouraging their employees to join health plans (Ellwood & Lundberg 1996).

Care networks and managed care may take one of many forms (Monaco & Goldschmidt 1997); these include:

- Health maintenance organisations (HMOs): an organisation that provides a defined range of health services to an individual (or group) for a specified period (usually a year) in exchange for a prospective (usually monthly) per capita (or per family) subscription payment.
- Independent practitioner association (IPA): an entity that enters into an arrangement for the provision of healthcare services with licensed medical practitioners and other healthcare providers, often for the purpose of contracting with MCOs to deliver services to their enrolees.
- Preferred provider organisation (PPO): an MCO that contracts with providers to deliver specified healthcare services to a defined population (enrolees) at a discount. A PPO usually has the following characteristics: discounted provider fees in exchange for a guaranteed volume of patients; monetary incentives for enrolees to use preferred network providers and broad-based utilisation management programmes.

## The success of managed-care networks

Increasingly the literature being reported in the USA is emphasising the positive impact of managed care on health and the economy. The pressures on healthcare services in the UK make NHS reform an increasing priority of healthcare policy-makers. In light of the success of managed care in the USA, it would appear that, if handled properly, managed care could produce substantial benefits for patients in the UK with improvements in quality of care and the introduction of new services.

Managed care has been successful because it brings together clinicians, managers and purchasers to establish needs and determine best practice in the management of patients. Comparative evaluation of alternative courses of management for specific groups of patients will reveal treatments, which are relatively ineffective, or too expensive, for the degree of benefit they produce.

## Managed care and cancer

One of the disease areas that was initially perceived as being particularly vulnerable to the changes in healthcare delivery brought about by MCOs was cancer care. Managed care has a particularly large impact on cancer care: research and clinical trials, practitioner training, prevention and early detection, treatment decisions, palliation and psychological support, and timely referral to hospices (Simmons & Goldforth

1997). It is important to appreciate the cost of cancer care in the managed-care setting given MCOs' emphasis on cost containment. Despite a level of incidence little more than half that of cardiovascular disease, cancer care generates $US10 billion more in annual treatment costs in the USA (Simmons & Goldforth 1997) than does spending on cardiovascular care.

The gold standard of cancer care consists of a specifically tailored treatment programme for the patient, composed of appropriate screening, diagnostic tests, standard and new treatments and, increasingly, participation in well-designed clinical trials. Referral to clinical trials is considered the standard of care when patients have exhausted proven treatment options or when those options are inappropriate (Monaco & Goldschmidt 1997). The main fear arising about managed care and its influence over cancer care is that treatment options may be taken away from the patient/ oncologist partnership in favour of a one-size-fits-all system of cancer care (Monaco & Goldschmidt 1997). However, the oncology community must change with the times, removing impediments of inefficient, unnecessary care, and become partners with MCOs to develop cancer care management systems that retain sufficient flexibility to accommodate individual patient requirements.

The ideal cancer programme within an MCO will include activities to help enrolees avoid cancer. Such a programme will promote early detection of cancer, enable access to best treatment and follow-up (over both the short and the long term) and monitor for late effects. The essential over-riding responsibility of the MCO is to help the enrolee lead a healthy, productive life. Managed care is much more capable of promoting wellness and prevention and early detection of cancer than the traditional fee-for-service medicine. This can be achieved by offering regular, periodic communications, providing health education to encourage wellness and prevention (e.g. promoting a healthy lifestyle and encouraging an annual mammogram), and offering preventive interventions such as smoking cessation programmes.

Compared with traditional fee-for-service medicine, MCOs can provide better access to medical advice and can manage demand for care more cost-effectively. Through health education MCOs will motivate patients to seek care and advice and, by providing greater access to screening and other preventive measures, MCOs should be able to detect and treat patients with cancer at earlier stages, greatly improving survival rates. With early detection, MCOs may also reduce the need in some cancer cases for costly therapies.

Encouraging literature concerning managed care and its effect on cancer care is emerging in original scientific articles as well as on the internet and in the media. The editorial by Berman in *The Seattle Times* 'Managed care saves lives in Washington' gives a positive insight into cancer patients' opinions on managed care, reporting that MCOs' comprehensive health plans provide patients with 'high-quality', life-saving, managed care. The author concludes that the health of millions of Washington State residents is improving and healthcare inflation has slowed, allowing more people access to health coverage (Berman 1998).

Bennett *et al.* (1997) carried out an analysis of case studies of approaches to prostate cancer by MCOs, and a survey of corporate medical directors at large MCOs. The authors concluded that prostate cancer is a feasible area for development and evaluation of population-based approaches to cancer care by MCOs. They believe that MCOs have the potential to improve clinical care and outcomes for large numbers of men with prostate cancer.

In summary MCOs that are committed to patient care should have accountability for results, cost containment, measurement of outcomes, health promotion and disease prevention programmes, resource consumption management, emphasis on primary care and continuous quality improvement (Monaco & Goldschmidt 1997). Managed care, therefore, may be very beneficial to NHS reform, the only caveat remaining that increasing cost pressures may result in the unintended consequence of diminishing quality of care, thus the need to assess quality of care and its change over time with the introduction of reform.

## Managed-care networks and pharmaceuticals

Managed-care organisations have a mandate for providing high-quality care while at the same time controlling costs. As a result of the growing prevalence of such organisations and the increasing likelihood that they provide prescription benefits coverage, it is not surprising that managed care has scrutinised drug budgets for areas of potential cost savings. In 1997 managed care was responsible for more than 50% of the drug market volume (BCG 1993). It is now estimated that MCOs are responsible for 90% of the drug market volume (BCG 1993). Thus, the cost of drugs and the value that drugs provide to managed-care networks has become of great importance. Although it is acknowledged that pharmaceuticals are only a fraction of the overall MCO budget (Sclar & Skaer 1992), in recent years the cost of pharmaceutical products has risen faster than the overall inflation rate (Tanouye 1996). MCOs have used a variety of techniques to control expenditure on pharmaceuticals (Cohen 1996):

- Formularies: lists of selected pharmaceuticals for prescribers
- Drug utilisation review: monitoring prescribing habits
- Generic substitution: replacing branded prescriptions with generics wherever possible
- Therapeutic substitution: use of least expensive patented product in the same class
- Reduced distribution costs: use of mail order and discount outlets
- Pharmacy benefits managers: one management system for distribution and utilisation strategies.

The attempt by MCOs to manage healthcare costs has led to an important shift in emphasis, whereby the prescriber is no longer the sole decision-maker in the process of treatment and the payer is becoming increasingly influential in the prescription decision. This has created a new challenge for the pharmaceutical industry, which must no longer demonstrate simply the clinical value of their drugs but also their economic value.

## The pharmaceutical industry and managed care

The emergence of managed-care networks has encouraged a shift within the pharmaceutical industry to emphasise the overall value of a product rather than simply concentrating on the acquisition price. The demonstration of economic value has led to many firms establishing pharmacoeconomic or outcomes research divisions (Stewart 1989; Pollard 1990) and has also seen an increasing use of pharmacoeconomic evaluations. Pharmacoeconomics has been defined (Bootman 1995) as the best method to 'describe and analyse costs and consequences of pharmaceuticals and pharmaceutical services and their impact on individuals, health care systems, and society'. In other words, any products that provide effective interventions for patients should not be judged solely on their purchase price.

Pharmacoeconomics is a valuable tool for obtaining information on the value of pharmaceuticals (Dragaulis & Coons 1995), but like any tool it is only useful if people can understand, believe and use the data that it produces.

## Adding value: partnership between the pharmaceutical industry and managed-care networks

It is sometimes felt (Murray & Deardorff 1998) that managed-care networks and the pharmaceutical companies have interests that are in total conflict. In fact they do have a large area of common ground, which is the investigation of the effects of pharmaceutical products on the total healthcare costs of patients. However, achieving better results for patients will require a partnership approach between the industry and MCOs in which the role of pharmacoeconomics will be crucial.

One of the major barriers to the use of pharmacoeconomics within managed-care settings is caused by the organisational arrangements of many MCOs. Until relatively recently, most MCOs had budget and accountability systems that encouraged the minimisation of costs within specified departments. This narrow focus encouraged an approach that rewarded the control of pharmacy costs and created the illusion that using the cheapest possible drug treatment among a selection of alternatives was the best approach (Draugalis & Coons 1995; Murray & Deardorff 1998). Such systems have begun to change as MCOs have shifted to a more organisational approach, and considered the impact of acquiring more expensive drugs that can be shown to offset the higher costs of disease exacerbation.

Resulting from managed health care, the pharmaceutical industry is no longer able to sell products based solely on safety and clinical efficacy. For both historical and regulatory reasons, many of the studies that pharmaceutical companies conducted as part of the approval of the US Food and Drugs Administration (FDA) process were of limited practical interest to the MCO industry. Research often involved comparisons with placebo, under strict control with rigid criteria for inclusion or exclusion. This served to eliminate a large segment of the MCO patient population, who where part of the audience for new medications. Cost data were also questionable in that costs may well be protocol driven and considered over too short a duration.

Meanwhile, the most commonly accepted way of MCOs collecting data on a new drug is through a formal study where individuals are randomised to receive either the new drug or the usual care drug. Resource utilisation, quality of life, patient satisfaction and overall cost can be measured and compared. These studies provide MCOs with just the material to allow them to make informed coverage decisions. Although a relatively limited number of studies have been conducted in the MCO setting, the lack of MCO research involvement should not be confused with a lack of interest in study results.

Many MCO decision-makers have become increasingly sophisticated in scrutinising the quality of published reports on the value of new drugs. Yet, given their lack of infrastructure and research skills, it makes great sense for MCOs to partner with the more experienced research organisations such as those at pharmaceutical companies. Despite different business priorities, there is potential similarity in research interests, particularly that of outcome assessment. A win–win situation can definitely be created when these areas of overlapping interest are exploited. The combination can provide MCOs with the relevant skills needed to conduct outcomes research. Pharmaceutical companies can then use these data from these studies to demonstrate the value of their new products. Indeed, pharmaceutical companies already need this information to support their marketing projects.

Previous barriers to why research collaborations had not existed included the following.

## From managed care

- A sense of this not being part of MCO mission
- Scepticism of drug companies' motives
- Lack of understanding of design issues
- MCO restrictions on experimental drugs and procedures for members (FDA mandates, etc.).

## From pharmaceutical companies

- Cost of research with managed care adds to already huge clinical trial costs
- A tradition of having worked with academia and private centres with research expertise
- Scepticism that MCOs want free drugs/money with no interest in research
- Need to conduct research to FDA regulations and mandates.

Commentators such as Tugwell (1996) and Drummond (1995) have articulated the need for efforts to raise the level of consciousness about the importance of usual care outcome studies. The partnership of industry and managed care should advance the knowledge of practice patterns, relevant outcomes, costs and quality-of-life considerations for various treatments. Generally, the research community will benefit from the lessons learned by conducting a clinical trial in a more realistic general practice environment. MCOs stand to gain a better understanding of the complexities and restraints involved in conducting clinical research, potentially increasing their knowledge of how and why manufacturers present information to them. Manufacturers will in turn gain a better understanding of the efficiencies and goals of quality patient care provided in a managed-care setting. This will assist manufacturers in creating more meaningful messages for managed-care providers. The usual care trial offers MCOs the information to make informed decisions. Manufacturers are optimistic that, with information gained through the usual care trial, they will confirm that the information received was credible, relevant and necessary to make formulary decisions. The important issue is to strike a balance between marketplace needs and the expense and time involved in conducting large-scale, usual care trials. This matter needs continual assessment to develop maximum mutual benefit.

Pharmaceutical outcomes research offers the MCO a tool to increase financial competitiveness and a means to demonstrate the overall value of the healthcare benefit package to its members. MCOs, in return, can do much to facilitate outcomes research. Of particular importance should be a commitment to build, enhance and standardise their databases, making them more accessible to researchers from both pharmaceutical firms and universities.

Overcoming the technical and organisational barriers to collaboration between MCOs and external researchers will require concerted effort. The various parties involved should develop trust, recognise common ground, share risk, promote communication and design research sensitive to MCO objectives.

Looking to the future, one major challenge to address is the potential for bias and conflict of interest in the conduct of health outcomes research projects and the reporting of results. The results of outcomes projects have a significant impact on formulary and clinical decisions; so the validity, reproducibility and trustworthiness of these results must stand close public scrutiny. In addition, outcomes research is pretty much in its infancy and many of the methods employed are controversial. It certainly seems that transparent presentation of data is the most widely accepted criterion for judging the quality and credibility of published study results. The pharmaceutical industry has monetary resources and needs information for product and promotion decisions. The managed-care industry has data sets but is short on resources to design studies and analyse data. Collaboration must be viewed as the route to success.

## Disease management

As MCOs begin to take a more organisational and system-wide approach to healthcare delivery there has been an increasing recognition that a comprehensive, multidisciplinary, collaborative approach to healthcare delivery and prevention is therefore essential as the complexity of health problems increases. Such an approach may take the form of 'disease management'. The three main components of disease management are:

- A knowledge base defining the natural history of a disease, and guidelines regarding the care to be provided, by whom and in what setting
- A healthcare delivery system made up of partnerships between primary care providers through to pharmaceuticals
- A continuous improvement process measuring and evaluating clinical, financial, satisfaction and health status outcomes, thereby continually ensuring the highest quality of care.

Providers of health care need to work in partnership with pharmaceutical companies to manage the process of care, to ensure patients are involved in healthcare decisions and to understand their treatment. In working closely with the pharmaceutical industry, healthcare providers can ensure that treatments are used appropriately and patients comply better with the planned therapy. The pharmaceutical industry is well positioned to play a key role in managing cancer and other serious and costly diseases as the industry can contribute significantly to MCOs by:

- continuing to create medical breakthroughs
- collaborating with MCOs to help control costs
- educating the physician, the pharmacists and other providers, strengthening the provider–patient relationship and improving patient compliance to drug regimens.

Through their expert knowledge of diseases including cancer, the pharmaceutical industry can help support cost management. Provision of therapeutic cost-effectiveness data, development of information on outcomes and trends measurement, support of protocol development for further therapeutic research, and development of delivery systems and dosage regimens (enhancing compliance) are all important cost-containment strategies performed by pharmaceuticals.

Pharmaceutical companies are increasing the number of employees with specific responsibility for managed care (BCG 1993), and are incorporating the needs of managed care in planning product development. It is hoped that, by developing expertise in health economics, pharmaceuticals can bring the benefit of that expertise to healthcare providers, as well as expertise in educating prescribers and patients and in organising healthcare initiatives.

# Conclusions

In summary, managed care can encourage and enable people to lead healthier, more productive lives, and can improve cost-effectiveness of cancer care through better education, self-care and prevention programmes. Managed care can also provide more efficient diagnosis and management of chronic diseases, producing better survival rates and long-term care. The pharmaceutical industry is well positioned to work in partnership with managed-care organisations and networks to explore the common ground and continue to deliver benefits to patients.

## *References*

Baronas AMK (1995). Partnering to provide high quality, cost-effective care for Medicaid/Medicare populations: affiliation strategies for providers and suppliers. Presentation to 'Capturing the emerging Medicaid/Medicare Managed Care Market for the Pharmaceutical Industry'. December 13, 14 Washington DC

Bennett CL *et al.* (1997). Approaches to prostate cancer by managed care organisations. *Urology* **50**(1), 79–86

Berman HS (1998). Managed care saves lives in Washington. *The Seattle Times* 30 April

Bootman JL (1995). Pharmacoeconomics and outcomes research. *American Journal of Health Systems Pharmacy* **52**(suppl), S16–S19

The Boston Consulting Group, Inc. (BCG) (1993). *The Changing Environment for US Pharmaceuticals: The role of pharmaceutical companies in a systems approach to health care*. Boston, MA: The Boston Consulting Group

Cohen KR (1996). Managed competition: implications for the US pharmaceutical industry. *Journal of Research in Pharmacy and Economics* **7**, 29–40

Dragaulis JR & Coons SJ (1995). Pharmacoeconomic research – facilitating collaboration among academic institutions, managed care organisations, and the pharmaceutical industry: a conference report. *Clinical Therapeutics* **17**, 89–108

Drummond M (1995). Economic analysis alongside clinical trials: Problems and potential. *Journal of Rheumatology* **22**, 1403–1407

Ellwood PM Jr & Lundberg GD (1996). Managed care: a work in progress. *Journal of the American Medical Association* **276**, 1083–1087

Krumholz HM (1999). Managed care and quality of care. *Journal of General Internal Medicine* **14**(2), 136–137

Monaco GP & Goldschmidt P (1997). What is proper cancer care in the era of managed care? *Oncology* **11**(1), 65–78

Muirhead G (1996). Prescription drug use rising among Medicare enrollees. *Drug Topics* 19 February, 66

Murray MD & Deardorff FW (1998). Does managed care fuel pharmaceutical industry growth? *Pharmacoeconomics* **14**, 341–348

Pollard MR (1990). Managed care and a changing pharmaceutical industry. *Health Affairs* **9**, 55–65

Sclar DA & Skaer TL (1992). Pharmaceutical formulation and healthcare expenditures. *Pharmacoeconomics* **3**, 267–269

Simmons WJ & Goldforth L (1997) The impact of managed care on cancer care. *Cancer Practice* **5**, 111–118

Stewart JH (1989). Marketing to managed care institutions. *Drug Information Journal* **23**, 641–645

Tanouye E (1996). Although inflation is barely breathing, drug prices are showing stronger pulse. *Wall Street Journal* 15 February, A3

Tudor C (1999). Medicare, managed care, and cancer. *Oncology* **13**(5A), 191–194

Tugwell P (1996) Economic evaluation of the management of pain in osteoarthritis. *Drugs* **52**(suppl 3), 48–58

# Chapter 4

# Managed clinical networks: an example from cancer services

*James W Rimmer*

## Introduction

This chapter looks at the application of managed clinical networks to cancer services in the NHS in England and Wales. It highlights an example of a cancer network in the south west of England (Avon, Somerset and Wiltshire Cancer Services), and details how the views of patients and carers can be placed at the heart of service developments.

## Improving cancer services

The drive to improve cancer services in the National Health Service (NHS) in England and Wales has been driven by two key policy documents – the Calman–Hine Report (1995) and *The NHS Cancer Plan* (Department of Health 2000). These two policy documents have led a variety of innovations and re-design of cancer services, but the notion of managed clinical networks has been at the heart of these improvements.

## ASWCS: an example of a cancer network

Avon, Somerset and Wiltshire Cancer Services (ASWCS) is a network of NHS trusts and health authorities working together to improve cancer services. ASWCS was designated as one of four cancer networks in the south west by a Regional Office Review, which took place in December 1998 and was reported by the Regional Office in April 1999 (NHS Executive South & West 1999).

ASWCS covers a population of 2.1 million people and co-ordinates cancer care via a network of 14 site-specialist tumour groups and one palliative care group. The purpose of ASWCS is to improve the quality of cancer services through the delivery of the National Cancer Plan and the implementation of the recommendations in the Calman–Hine Report, and through local collaboration and partnership.

### Membership

Membership of ASWCS is made up of eight NHS trusts: East Somerset, Taunton & Somerset, Weston Area Healthcare, United Bristol Healthcare (UBHT), North Bristol, Royal United Hospital Bath (RUH), Swindon & Marlborough and Salisbury Health Care; three health authorities: Avon, Somerset and Wiltshire; and 14 primary care organisations (PCOs).

Two of the trusts within ASWCS provide radiotherapy services (UBHT and RUH) and two trusts (Swindon & Marlborough and Salisbury Health Care) look on the whole to cancer centres outside the ASWCS collaboration for their radiotherapy services (to Oxford and Southampton, respectively). In addition ASWCS covers approximately 60 cancer-specific voluntary sector organisations and groups.

## Structure

ASWCS is organised via a series of working groups, committees and projects (Figure 4.1). The work is co-ordinated by a small team of staff who are based in a central office.

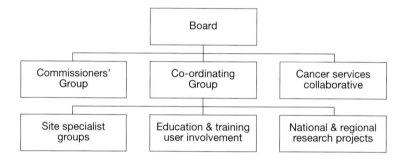

**Figure 4.1** Structure of ASWCS.

## ASWCS Board

The ASWCS Board consists of the chief executives or their director level representatives from each of the member organisations. Each health community also sends a PCO representative. The Board provides a strategic framework for cancer services across the three health communities.

## Co-ordinating Group

The Co-ordinating Group is chaired by the ASWCS lead clinician. The group shares good practice across ASWCS and implements the decisions of the Board. Each member organisation is represented by their lead cancer clinician and their lead cancer manager. Other organisations are also included: PCOs are represented by each health community; the voluntary sector and hospice movement are fully involved; and, patients and carers have a standing item on the agenda and have statutory membership through a user involvement group.

## Site specialist groups

Each cancer tumour has its own site specialist group. In total ASWCS has 14 tumour groups and a non-tumour-specific palliative care group. The role of these site specialist groups is to develop standards of care and to share good practice. Many, although not all, of these groups include user views, obtained through a variety of methods. These range from users sitting as group members, to user surveys and focus groups.

## Commissioners' Group

The three health authorities also meet to develop common commissioning policies across ASWCS. Examples of issues at which this Group looks are: high-cost cancer drugs through a Drug Policy Forum, and the equity of chemotherapy and radiotherapy services across ASWCS. The challenge currently facing the Commissioners' Group is how to involve PCOs more actively.

## Work groups

ASWCS also supports a range of core subgroups looking at: research and development, user involvement, education and training, and the cancer services collaborative.

### Research and development

ASWCS is one of the nine phase I networks in the National Cancer Research Network. This work started in April 2001 and will enable ASWCS to develop an infrastructure of research nurses and data managers across the network. The aims of the cancer network are, first, to double the number of cancer patients entered into trials by March 2003, and, second, to ensure that all patients across the network have the same opportunity to be entered into trials independent of where they are receiving their care.

### User involvement

The ASWCS User Involvement Group is a well-established group in ASWCS and has been in place in one form or another since 1997. The Group meets three or four times a year with the aim of providing a patient and carer perspective to the work undertaken by ASWCS. Members of the User Involvement Group attend the Co-ordinating Group to ensure that their views are represented and to contribute to the broader debate. ASWCS also has a Department of Health-funded research programme in user involvement which is looking at the best way to involve users in developing and evaluating cancer services. This is running from October 1999 to September 2002, working with the University of the West of England and the University of Warwick.

*Education and training*

The Education and Training Group looks to support cancer education across the network. The Group has focused on developing innovative methods of education and has received two research grants: one to develop an interprofessional cancer education programme and one to develop and evaluate training on user involvement for healthcare professionals.

*Cancer Services Collaborative*

ASWCS was also a phase I network for the Cancer Services Collaborative (October 1999 to March 2001). This work is continuing in phase II (April 2001 onwards) and will cover the following tumour sites: breast, lung, colorectal, upper gastrointestinal, gynaecological and urological. The aim of the Cancer Services Collaborative is to encourage cancer teams to improve the quality of the care that they are giving by focusing on the pathway of care that a patient follows. Quality improvement techniques are used to help teams to make changes and measure their impact.

## Summary of the ASWCS network

ASWCS is a proactive and innovative cancer network and is well respected for the work it has done in developing the agenda for cancer networks. ASWCS takes a developmental and collaborative approach to improving cancer services, and applies project work directly to service delivery, in order to ensure that programmes of work remain practical and based on the needs of cancer services. The cancer network works not just across trusts, PCOs and health authorities, but also with the academic community, the voluntary sector and local user groups.

## Involving patients and carers

Improving the quality of cancer services is a high priority for the NHS. The Calman–Hine Report stressed the importance of involving user views to evaluate and develop services (for the purpose of this chapter the term 'users' has been used to mean patients and carers, i.e. direct users of cancer services). More recently, the White Papers – *The New NHS* (NHS Executive 1997a) and *A First Class Service* (NHS Executive 1997b) – repeated the recommendation to involve users in the development of the NHS. ASWCS responded to this recommendation by forming a project group to develop user involvement for cancer services.

## Formation of a user involvement group

The development of user involvement in ASWCS is ongoing and it has had its fair share of positive developments, as well as more challenging difficulties. User involvement can prove a real test. The NHS has tended to focus on 'doing' user involvement rather than thinking about how it has been, or could be, done (Wedderburn-Tate 1994).

This chapter highlights some of the ways in which user involvement has taken place within ASWCS to date, what it has already achieved and what the hopes are for the future of user involvement.

In 1997, when ASWCS was formed, one of its first actions was to set up a group called the Patient Consultation Group, the purpose of which was to consider the user perspective for cancer services. The group was composed of healthcare professionals from a variety of backgrounds, including clinicians, nurses, managers, psychologists and public health doctors. The original aim of the Patient Consultation Group was to try to help cancer services to develop ways of involving the users of those services, and in a manner that would be clear and transparent. The group was facilitated by a senior clinician. This need for strong clinical leadership was recommended in the Department of Health (1999) guidelines and is supported by research evidence (Thomson *et al.* 2000). The group was supported by a range of members, many of whom had many years of experience of working with users to develop health services.

In April 1998, the Patient Consultation Group set itself two tasks (Patient Consultation Project Group 1998): first, to develop the mechanism by which patients and their carers can contribute to the development of site-specific cancer care protocols and, second, to establish the method of user consultation on completed protocols and service development plans.

The first set of site-specific cancer care standards at which this group attempted to look were the ASWCS Standards for Breast Cancer. They were keen to gain a user perspective in the consideration of these standards, although they struggled with how and/or when to bring users into the group. This issue was taken forward when one of the members decided to ask each member of the group to 'buddy' a woman who had had breast cancer. This was a useful start but had its own difficulties as highlighted in the data below.

In November 1998, ASWCS ran a conference for cancer service users and healthcare professionals – 'Improving Communication between Cancer Services Users and Health Care Professionals'. The conference hoped to achieve two aims: to help ASWCS develop an agenda focused on the needs of users of cancer services, and to recruit more patients and carers into the area of user involvement. In the first instance, the conference identified two major requirements for user involvement to develop. First, the conference highlighted the importance of an equal partnership between users and healthcare professionals and, second, it identified the need to instigate a development programme for cancer services users, to enable them to contribute effectively to service development and planning (Cancer Services User Involvement Group 1998). After this conference, a second complementary/competing user group was started – the User Involvement Group. The role of this new group and its relationship to the old Patient Consultation Group were blurred.

This new User Involvement Group again had the involvement of clinicians but was more obviously driven by the users and voluntary sector. Some confusion occurred for a period of time while both the Patient Consultation Group and the User Involvement Group coexisted. The membership lists of the two groups did have some overlap, but on the whole their memberships were different. The Patient Consultation Group had remained largely dominated by health service members and the User Involvement Group was largely dominated by users and the voluntary sector.

## Aims of user involvement

These two groups therefore had different but complementary aims. There was, however, confusion between the roles and the overlap between the two groups. To try to resolve some of this confusion the two groups met together in March 1999 and decided to merge to become the ASWCS User Involvement Group.

The aim for the newly merged and re-formed User Involvement Group was to ensure that user views are considered at every stage of the development of cancer services. This has been defined more recently as a mission statement, which states that the User Involvement Group aims 'To provide a supportive framework to encourage and enable users to influence ASWCS in improving provision, development and delivery of cancer services' (ASWCS Coordinating Group Minutes 2000, unpublished).

The membership of the group consists of cancer service users (defined by the group as patients and carers), healthcare professionals (doctors, nurses and managers) and members from the voluntary sector. It aims to have these three groupings represented in equal numbers.

## Review of user involvement in the network

An action research study was undertaken to evaluate the effectiveness of the User Involvement Group and to assess to what extent the involvement of users in the cancer network led to change (Rimmer 2000). Excerpts of the data are given below.

## The action research framework

Data are reviewed against the typologies for action research developed by Hart and Bond (1995, pp 40–43). Hart and Bond devised four action research typologies – experimental, organisational, professionalising and empowering. This chapter focuses on the typology of empowerment. The data examine the key areas in which the User Involvement Group was looking to bring about change and assess to what extent these changes were effected.

### Education and training

Education and training are crucial to the development of user involvement for a managed clinical network. ASWCS worked closely with Cancerlink to develop a joint 2-day training programme for both users and healthcare professionals. The data suggest that participants both identified increased personal confidence and highlighted a raised awareness of both their needs and the needs of others.

Members were very clear, for example, of the benefits brought about by the training sessions which were run for members of the User Involvement Group:

> The Cancerlink workshops made a hell of a difference. And at the end of it, you've actually got users who can work with site specialist teams with confidence.

> IV-1b, voluntary sector

The benefit of raising the consciousness of the group was also recognised. Members recognised that, although they might not yet have delivered a great deal of change in terms of service delivery, people were now more aware of them and their role. This raised awareness applies as much to the increased understanding of individuals within the group, as it does to the broader community whom the group is trying to serve and influence:

> I mean it's good, it's good for people who go, because we learn things and discuss things and as a general raising the level, raising awareness

> FG-1a, user

The group were aware, however, that they were perhaps giving expression to the views of those in society who, to a certain extent, already had a voice, i.e. middle-class women, but were failing to empower or represent the views of less powerful groups – people with low socioeconomic status or ethnic minorities:

> I have been going to a cancer support group in Knowle West . . . it's a very old estate, very working class estate. And I've been to a group of the estate, from the estate . . . and they've got all the same issues about cancer that all of us have. But they don't get expressed, you see.

> FG-1a, user

Finally, although there was some debate about who set the agenda for the group – the government, the ASWCS team or the users. It was noted that the goal of the group was to work towards an agenda arising out of the needs of the users. Progress towards this enhances the role of the users on the group:

> Calman says we have to develop services and they've got to be patient-centred. So, there is an agenda, and I'm always concerned about what I call the government NHS agenda squashing the possibility of the agenda arising from the patient.

> IV-1b, voluntary sector

## Development of the group

Hart and Bond acknowledge the importance of interaction between group members in achieving their goals. They suggest that this is particularly demonstrated through the membership arrangements displayed by different groups: experimental action research groups have a fixed membership, organisational groups a selected membership, professionalising groups a shifting membership, and empowering groups a fluid membership.

The User Involvement Group demonstrates a variation across Hart and Bond's action research typologies for this criterion. Although there is a fixed overall membership of about 30 (experimental), the numbers and individuals attending any one meeting can vary (empowering): the average attendance at regular group meetings was about 15 (i.e. half the total membership). Some members felt that they had been selected (organisational) whereas others recognised that the Group had started as a group of healthcare professionals but had shifted over time to be more balanced with users and the voluntary sector:

> The membership is a mixture of health care professionals and patients, users.
>
> FG-1a, user

## Problem focused

A problem-focused approach in action research can be defined as identifying issues that need changing. The User Involvement Group identified several key areas over the period of the group. These issues varied over the period of study with the group.

Initially the group recognised that there needed to be a slow process of group development: some of the issues that had arisen from merging the Patient Consultation Group and the User Involvement Group needed to be resolved. This was particularly true of the power balance between the user members and the healthcare members. The empowering typology suggests that the definitions of these problems should be negotiated. Initially the group focused on issues identified by the healthcare professionals, and only more latterly on issues raised by the group themselves. There continues to be tension between meeting the needs of the group and those of the NHS:

> I'm always concerned about what I call the government NHS agenda squashing the possibility of the agenda arising from the patient.
>
> IV-1b, voluntary sector

Over time, the problems that the User Involvement Group have focused on have changed to meet the needs of the user members:

> So we said no, go back to the organisers, we want to be in the morning on the agenda, by all means give us a slot in the afternoon as well. And [an ASWCS team member] went back and got it.
>
> FG-3b, user

Increasingly, the Group have also had the opportunity to identify specific problems that they have experienced as individuals and these have been taken up by members of the ASWCS team. A protocol for this was developed and agreed by the User Involvement Group in July 1999 which has proved a useful way of solving these specific issues:

> And, yeah, having lost someone, I know some of the problems that are associated
>
> FG-3b, user

## Change intervention

Although action research focuses on change, the changes achieved by the User Involvement Group may not be as discrete and identifiable as one would hope. An example of this is the aim of the User Involvement Group to raise their profile. An experimental framework would enable some measurable evidence of a raised profile, such as the number of formal ASWCS meetings at which members were represented. An empowering framework, however, allows for softer evidence of a raised profile. An example of this is a user member's comment about how the group was now perceived:

> It is hard to say exactly what has changed, but I think, as I said before, people know we are about and . . . that we are likely to challenge or pick up on things.
>
> FG-4b, user

The basis of change may also be more in the process of change rather than in the intervention itself. The User Involvement Group could identify practical examples, such as user involvement in the ASWCS process of accrediting cancer services, but members also acknowledged that changes were to some degree evolutionary:

> . . . because things take time. Things don't change overnight. Things tend to evolve as well.
>
> FG-3a, user

Changes in process are also a key feature of the empowering typology. When members of the User Involvement Group attended a research seminar held in February 2000, members were asked to consider the problem of measuring satisfaction with user involvement. This issue had not been raised by members of the group; it was under discussion to meet the needs of the Department of Health User Involvement Research Project. Although the meeting was not on that occasion evaluated, the author's notes suggest that it is unlikely to have met the needs of the users who attended, focusing as it did purely on the needs of the research team. This was reflected on by the research team and it was agreed to provide a more balanced approach to future seminars where the needs for both users and researchers could be identified and met.

## Improvement and involvement

Improvement and involvement are crucial when evaluating the involvement of groups of individuals in health and social care. Hart and Bond (1995, p 54) state that the aim of user involvement is to 'improve professional practice for the benefit of users of a service and to involve those concerned in the process of change'. The User Involvement Group presented a clear case where the intention had been to involve them in an empowering manner. The ASWCS Breast Site Specialist Group had intended to ask the User Involvement Group to help them develop standards for the care of breast cancer patients:

> We had come together to work out how best to give support to site specialist groups
> for user involvement
>
> FG-5a, NHS manager

. . . but the reality had been that instead of involvement from the outset, as the empowerment typology would support, the group had been presented with a set of pre-written standards for comment:

> . . . and then, during this work we basically got presented with a fully written up
> standards.
>
> FG-5a, NHS manager

This behaviour is that identified under the professionalising typology. Thus, although a group might set out to work in an empowering manner, when measured against defined criteria some behaviours can be seen to fall outside that typology. Other actions, such as the group's involvement in the accreditation process, fall more clearly into the empowering typology, where the areas for improvement were identified by both healthcare professionals and user members:

> And there have been some accreditations done recently, where users have
> been involved.
>
> FG-4b, user

## Cyclic process

The notion of cyclical processes is not uncommon in health care, with examples being clinical audit and reflective practice. These processes have also been useful ways of involving users in the development and evaluation of healthcare services (Kelson 1997).

The empowering definition of the cyclic process suggests that cycles should be open-ended and process driven. Clear examples of this style are found in comments from members, although sometimes there can be a fine line between a process being open-ended and lacking direction:

> I think process is very important
>
> FG-1a, user

. . . sometimes I have thought, 'where are we going?'

FG-4b, user

There was also a recognition that change is a complex process, and that the User Involvement Group needs to influence other groups in order to make changes. The ASWCS Co-ordinating Group was established to drive the cancer agenda forward in hospitals and health authorities. The User Involvement Group state clearly the need to influence this group:

> For example we are present and on the agenda at the co-ordinating group, which is quite an important group

FG-4b, user

## Summary of user views

The ASWCS User Involvement Group, although having some failings, can clearly be demonstrated to have achieved its aim of developing cancer services. Although the reconfiguration of services is not always directly patient led, the role and profile of patients and carers as part of the managed care network have been demonstrated. As one member of the user involvement group stated:

> . . . the User Involvement Group 'has a rich history and I am glad you are writing it up . . . the motto should be try, try and try again, because something is obviously working very well now'.

W-1c, voluntary sector

## Conclusion

### Overview

Cancer services in England are being encouraged to form cancer networks to improve and co-ordinate services. Services must be developed to be user focused and a well-supported and -resourced user involvement programme can help to achieve this focus:

- Managed clinical networks are key to developing and improving cancer services.
- All sectors need to be involved at all levels in these networks.
- Networks do not appear over night – relationships and trust take time to develop.
- Service users can provide both support and encouragement to developing these services

### *References*

Calman K & Hine D (1995). *A Policy Framework for Commissioning Cancer Services: A report by the expert advisory group on cancer to the chief medical officers of England and Wales.* London: Department of Health & Welsh Office

Cancer Services User Involvement Group (1998). *Improving Communication between Cancer Services Users and Health Care Professionals.* Bristol: Cancer Services User Involvement Group

Department of Health (1999). *Patient and Public Involvement in the New NHS*. London: Department of Health

Department of Health (2000). *The NHS Cancer Plan*. London: HMSO

Hart E & Bond M (1995). *Action Research for Health and Social Care*. Buckingham: Open University Press

Kelson M (1997). *Promoting Patient Involvement in Clinical Audit*. London: College of Health

NHS Executive (1997a). *The New NHS: Modern, dependable*. Leeds: NHS Executive,

NHS Executive (1997b). *A First Class Service*. Leeds: NHS Executive

NHS Executive South & West (1999). *A Review of Cancer Services in the South and West*. Bristol: NHS Executive South & West

Patient Consultation Project Group (1998). *Role, Responsibilities and Accountability*. Bristol: Avon & Somerset Cancer Services

Rimmer J (2000). Does involving users in the development of cancer services lead to change? Oxford: University of Oxford, MSc Dissertation

Thomson O'Brien MA, Oxman AD, Haynes RB *et al*. (2000). Local opinion leaders: effects on professional practice and health care outcomes. *Cochrane Database System Review* (2) CD000125.

Wedderburn-Tate C (1994).User involvement – without the bruises. *Nursing Management* **1**, 10–11

Chapter 5

# The Salick Health Care experience in cancer disease management under the American system of managed care

*William Audeh*

## Introduction: Salick Health Care and cancer disease management

Salick Health Care (SHC) is an integrated network of cancer delivery sites, or cancer centres, affiliated with major hospitals around the USA. SHC Cancer Centers provide a full range of services for individuals with cancer and haematological disorders for whom specialised care is necessary. The comprehensive nature of these centres is evident in the services provided: screening, diagnosis, treatment, supportive care, and psychological and nutritional support. SHC has been operating since 1983, and currently has eight cancer centres located in the USA. It is estimated that 15,000–20,000 new cancer cases are seen each year within the SHC network, in addition to 250,000–300,000 patient visits. Over 100 physicians are affiliated with this network, including medical oncologists, radiation oncologists, surgical oncologists, gynaecological oncologists and pain management specialists. The centres are outpatient facilities, and many are open 24 hours a day in an effort to avoid unnecessary admissions to hospital and emergency room visits after hours. Clinical programmes within SHC Cancer Centers include state-of-the-art treatment protocols and technology, and active participation in clinical trials. The experience of co-ordinating the many aspects of cancer care within a single facility, and within a national network of facilities, led to the development of a comprehensive disease management approach to cancer care. It is the philosophy of SHC that a comprehensive disease management approach to cancer is needed to manage the complex clinical, social and psychological needs of the cancer patient, and provide the highest standard of care. In light of the fragmented healthcare system in the USA, patients in particular have embraced the SHC model of care, and patient satisfaction surveys have been consistently high. It is the goal of this chapter to describe the application of this model to the managed care system of healthcare delivery.

## The rise of managed care in the USA

The success of the SHC model of care, and expansion of the SHC network, took place during a period of enormous change in US health care. This change was characterised by the recognition of skyrocketing costs of health care, particularly cancer care, and a lack of willingness on the part of the public to pay these costs. Since 1990, cancer care has accounted for approximately 10% of all healthcare expenditure in the USA. Oncology drug costs have been rising at 35% per year, double the rate of other drug classes. In addition, in response to public demand and growing frustration with the lack of demonstrable progress in AIDS and cancer, the Food and Drug Administration (FDA) accelerated the drug approval process, opening the way for significant numbers of new and costly oncology drugs to enter the market. Cancer costs have risen dramatically during the 1990s, with direct costs of US$27 billion in 1990, rising to US$100 billion in 2000. Indirect costs, caused by morbidity, mortality and lost productivity resulting from cancer, were calculated at US$69 billion in 1990, and are likely to have been enormously higher in 2000.

In response to the rising costs of health care, managed care developed and grew in prominence during the early 1990s, primarily driven by the demands of employers for low-cost health care for their employees. Government-mandated provision of health insurance by employers led to demands for cost-containment as health care premiums rose to meet the rising costs of unrestricted healthcare delivery. In a survey of employers in the mid-1990s asking which factors determined choice of health plans, employers listed 'cost' as the number 1 factor. Of note is the fact that quality of care provided by health plans, in the form of 'clinical outcomes', ranked a distant seventh in importance (Reynolds 1999).

As a method for containing or reducing costs of health care, managed care has been quite effective and, as a result, by 1998, over 25% of the US population was covered by a managed care plan. This included private employers as well as government-funded programmes, in which managed care plans managed the care of 43% of Medicaid enrolees, and 30% of Medicare enrolees, or over 70 million Americans (Mighion *et al.* 1999). Managed care is primarily associated with the health maintenance organisation (HMO), in which the greatest control is exerted over the activities of physicians, nurses, hospitals and patients. Under this system, the choice of physicians to whom a patient may have access is often restricted. Often the site of care, and the process by which a patient is cared for or referred to a specialist are tightly regulated, usually with guidelines intended to achieve cost-effectiveness, without, it is hoped, compromising quality of care. Some HMOs, such as the Kaiser–Permanente system, provide medical care by employing physicians, but this is the exception, and most health plans contract with private doctors and physician groups to provide care to their enrolees. The contract with the physicians may allow for the physicians to charge a fee for service, albeit at a discounted rate, although the most effective method for cost reduction is capitation.

In a capitation agreement, physicians are simply paid a small fee per member per month, placing the full financial risk and responsibility for providing care in the hands of the physicians. In regions in which HMOs have succeeded in capturing a large segment of the health coverage for a population, the results of this system may yield unintended consequences, such as inadequate care delivery or insufficient payment to physicians. The forces at play in the managed care system are summarised below:

- Government requires employers to provide health insurance
- Employers, in turn, demand reduced premiums from health plans
- Health plans reduce premiums competitively by effecting cost-control measures, including reducing fees paid to physicians through capitation contracts
- Physicians agree to deliver care within the limits of capitation, or risk losing access to patients, particularly in regions with significant penetration by HMOs.

This set of factors poses the risk of conflicting incentives, which do not reward, or reliably promote, the best patient care practices. Under this system, decision-making about how care is delivered is often controlled by the HMO, or left to the doctor when the doctor is bearing the financial risk within a capitated agreement. The HMO and/or physician must then balance cost-effectiveness and clinical benefit. If the decision is made in favour of cost-effectiveness, patient care may suffer. If cost is ignored, and patient care is the sole concern, physicians within capitated contracts may suffer enormous financial losses and bankruptcy, as was recently the case in California (*Los Angeles Times* 2000). Although this problem may be easily solved in simple and uncomplicated medical decision-making, it is fraught with difficulties when cancer care is concerned, given the complexity, high cost and rapid changes in the field. With the rise of managed care, the situation was ripe for negative outcomes for cancer patients.

Where cost containment has indeed been the primary goal, and without the application of specific expertise in cancer care, indiscriminate methods for cost control have been employed by some health plans, including:

- placing a daily limit on spending per patient, regardless of the clinical situation
- restricting access to specialists through gatekeepers
- restricting access to high-cost drugs.

Unintended consequences of such indiscriminate cost-containment measures are as follows: daily spending limits could be avoided by 'staggering' care by physicians, e.g. selecting multi-day chemotherapy instead of single-day regimens, substituting low-cost medications (such as antiemetics) for more efficacious high-cost drugs, and scheduling diagnostic studies and laboratory work on days separate from therapy (requiring multiple trips to hospital for frequently ill cancer patients). Restricted access to specialists, under the assumption that specialists are high utilisers of healthcare resources, led to the potential for inappropriate use of diagnostics by non-specialists (e.g. unnecessary and/or inappropriate biopsy and imaging tests for diagnosis and staging of cancer), or delayed and inadequate therapy for cancer-related problems. Restricted use of high-cost drugs, regardless of efficacy relative to lower-cost alternatives, also created the opportunity for inappropriate substitution and therapy below the standard of care.

In contradistinction to these methods for cost containment is the disease management approach, which attempts to identify opportunities for cost-effectiveness within the context of appropriate therapy and agreed standards of care. The disease management approach is based on the assumption that much of the avoidable cost of health care is the result of mismanagement of resources as a result of fragmentation of care and lack of communication between caregivers, and the undesirable outcomes of inappropriate clinical care, resulting in excess morbidity and mortality. The differences between these approaches to health care are summarised in Table 5.1.

**Table 5.1** Managed care versus disease management: definitions in the USA

| Managed care | Disease management |
|---|---|
| Episodic care delivery | Continuum of care |
| Goals:<br>    Cost minimisation<br>    Outcome data | Goals:<br>    Best patient outcomes<br>    Cost minimisation |
| Avoid specialist care | Multi-speciality co-ordination |
| Data collection:<br>    To monitor costs<br>    To meet NCQA requirements | Data collection:<br>    To measure outcomes<br>    To monitor costs |
| Minimal guidelines required | Broad clinical guidelines based on established standards of practice |

NCQA, National Committee for Quality Assurance.

Out of the SHC experience in the management of comprehensive outpatient cancer centres, a disease management approach to cancer care was developed. This expertise was then offered on a contractual basis to health plans such as HMOs, in care delivery sites geographically separate from SHC Cancer Centers. In this way, a 'virtual' cancer centre could be developed within a healthcare system, in which the necessary elements of comprehensive cancer care could be connected and utilised in a manner that consolidated or 'de-fragmented' care. The goals of applying oncology disease management to the HMO setting were to maintain or improve quality of care, while seeking opportunities for cost containment (based on knowledge derived from the SHC Cancer Center experience).

## Oncology disease management in managed care

In 1994, the first US contract to manage cancer care within a managed care system (oncology 'carve-out') was undertaken by SHC. A second contract soon followed and, over the course of 5 years, over 400,000 HMO enrolees were covered by SHC Oncology Disease Management, under the SHC subsidiary known as 'SalickNet'. These contracts with US HMOs involved a sharing of financial risk, with a capitated agreement based on a per member per month fee. From 1994 to 1999, SalickNet provided oncology disease management for over 10,000 cancer patients.

### The structure of SalickNet

SalickNet took a step-wise approach to managing cancer within a large managed healthcare system, summarised below:

- Establish clinical guidelines for the standard of care
- Assess the state of cancer care within the healthcare system
- Identify desired outcomes based on strengths and weaknesses of the healthcare system
- Develop relationship with physicians within the system
- Apply clinical guidelines with physician collaboration
- Collect data for measuring outcomes.

#### Clinical guideline development

Clinical guidelines were developed internally, using a variety of sources. An expert panel from all oncology specialities was convened for regular guideline development and updating sessions. These included medical oncology, radiation oncology, surgical oncology, radiology, nursing and pharmacy. The group used literature reviews by disease, as well as established guidelines from professional bodies such as the American Society of Clinical Oncology (ASCO), National Comprehensive Cancer Network (NCCN) and the Society of Surgical Oncology (SSO). As a result of the difficulties involved in the practical application of primary medical literature and written guidelines to actual patient care decision-making, all such data were organised into 'phases' of care: diagnosis, staging, therapy and follow-up. SHC guidelines were then developed at three levels of detail:

- Level I: disease-specific guidelines which included all phases of care for a particular disease.
- Level II: therapy-specific guidelines which focused on parameters for appropriate use of chemotherapy, radiation or surgery.
- Level III: agent-specific guidelines for the use of specific chemotherapy and supportive medications.

An example of this structure is as follows:

- Level I guideline: breast cancer.
- Level II guideline: adjuvant chemotherapy regimen, e.g. FAC (5-fluorouracil, Adriamycin [doxorubicin], cyclophosphamide).
- Level III guideline: use of doxorubicin (Adriamycin) or antiemetics.

## Assessing the state of the healthcare system

The application of guidelines to cancer care is complicated by the nature of the process of care delivery. The management of cancer involves multiple physicians in multiple sites, involved with the care of the patient over the course of a disease, which may vary from months to years. Unlike simple disease management approaches to episodic, self-limited disease events such as pneumonia or myocardial infarction, the disease management approach to cancer must reach across a spectrum of healthcare providers, and across time, through the phases of care.

In the typical healthcare system, the *diagnosis* of cancer is made by primary care physicians, surgeons or medical specialists such as pulmonologists or gastroenterologists, all of whom may utilise healthcare resources such as laboratory, imaging and medical procedures. Most healthcare systems do not define who is most responsible for *staging* of the newly diagnosed cancer patient. Patients are then referred for definitive therapy (and completion of staging) to radiation oncologists and/or medical oncologists. These practitioners also utilised additional laboratory and imaging studies, in addition to the application of therapy such as radiation, chemotherapy and supportive medications. After completion of therapy, patients may undergo periodic follow-up, with either the medical oncologist or the radiation oncologist, but more often through the original diagnosing physician, such as the primary care physician or surgeon. Again, in the follow-up period, there is great variability in the utilisation of laboratory and imaging studies to monitor for recurrence of disease. The following are evident from this process:

- Many physicians may be involved in the care of a single patient
- Considerable resources may be used by each physician in the course of caring for a cancer patient
- Quality of care as well as cost-effectiveness may be compromised during each phase of care.

Possible adverse consequences are:

- Diagnosis: delay in diagnosis may lead to more patients with an advanced, incurable stage of disease.

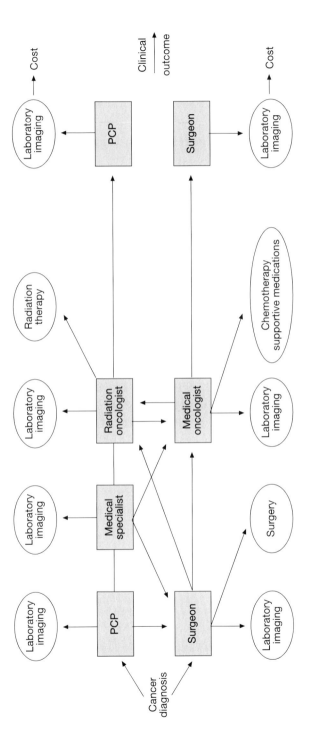

**Figure 5.1**  SalickNet: overview of cancer care network.

- Staging: inadequate staging will lead to inappropriate therapy, particularly unnecessary surgery and poor patient outcomes. Inappropriate staging may lead to overuse of resources and unnecessary procedures being performed.
- Therapy: lack of knowledge of the standard of care, or inadequate communication between physicians, can lead to missed opportunity for cure or better outcomes, particularly regarding cases in which combined modality therapy may be the optimal approach.
- Follow-up: inadequate monitoring for recurrence or treatment-related morbidity, or conversely excessive diagnostic evaluation, may lead to either poor long-term clinical outcomes or overuse of resources.

## Managing cancer care within a managed healthcare system

The challenge in managing the process of cancer care (cancer disease management) in the context of a healthcare system such as an HMO is to ensure that each component within the system is addressed in the clinical guidelines and is accessible by the 'managing team'. The managing team requires expertise in cancer, the ability to communicate with physicians and nurses within the system, and to collect data in the process. SalickNet organised a team of medical directors representing medical oncology, radiation oncology, surgical oncology and radiology, in addition to nurse case managers and clerical support staff for data collection. Information technology was developed to facilitate disease management, in the form of an interactive computer system, the Oncology Management, Assessment and Reporting (OMAR) system. This system contained the clinical guidelines in algorithmic or decision-tree format, and provided a mechanism for collecting data in real time, while maintaining record of the cost of care. Most importantly, the system allowed for collection of clinical outcome data.

The method by which the information was captured was based on prior authorisation for all elective or non-emergency care. The relationship between

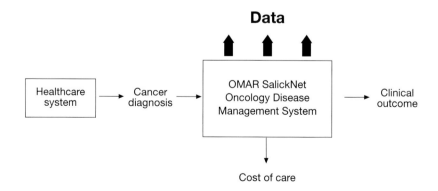

**Figure 5.2** SalickNet disease management system: data capture.

SalickNet and the physicians within the health plan imposed the requirement that all plans of care must be submitted to SalickNet in order for the physicians to be compensated (Figure 5.3). Although SalickNet accepted a capitated agreement with the HMO, the physicians were compensated by SalickNet on a discounted fee for service, thus removing the financial risk for physicians, and avoiding the conflicting incentives encountered by physicians when they are directly capitated.

Care plans for surgery, radiation and medical oncology were developed as paper forms that could be faxed or transmitted via computer. As payment to physicians was contingent on the timely submission of complete care plans (including diagnosis and stage), the quality and depth of the data were assured.

## Identifying desired outcomes

Key data elements were identified for maximising quality of care and determining opportunities for cost-effectiveness, including:

- Site of care delivery – outpatient vs inpatient
- Accuracy of diagnosis and staging (and avoidance of unnecessary surgery)
- Ensuring multidisciplinary approach to care
- Ensuring appropriate use of supportive medications.

The value of these elements is in reducing unnecessary diagnostic procedures, reducing unnecessary surgery and ensuring appropriate therapy for selected groups in which cure was possible, and in which deviation from the standard of care may compromise the chance of cure, such as adjuvant therapy for breast and colon cancer, and combined modality therapy approaches for certain advanced stage cancers such as breast, lung, colorectal, bladder, laryngeal and ovarian cancer.

### Data collection

Data collection included both clinical and financial data. Essential data such as a survey of cancer diagnoses were collected, as well as the costs associated with specific cancer types. For a particular diagnosis, such as breast cancer, the spectrum of stage at diagnosis offered the opportunity to assess the adequacy of screening, e.g. when an excess of breast cancer diagnosed at stages III and IV was noted in one healthcare system, it indicated an inadequate system for screening mammography and education about breast self-examination. This was reported to the health plan, which then instituted a policy of mailing and education for patients and primary care physicians.

### Site of care – reducing avoidable admission to hospital

It has been traditional to target hospital admission as a method of cost reduction. Admission to hospital for cancer patients is considered unnecessary if they involve

# SAMPLE FORM

**Phase of Care** (Check all that apply)
☐ Diagnosis
☐ Staging
☐ Therapy
☐ Follow-up

## RADIATION ONCOLOGY
### CLINICAL PLAN

**Urgency (check one)**
☐ Routine
☐ STAT

**GENERAL INFORMATION**

Member ID# _____ Member Name _____ (Last / First / Middle)
Physician Name _____ Facility Name _____
Diagnosis _____ Stage _____

**CLINICAL PLAN (Complete all areas that apply)** Anticipated Start Date: _____ Completion Date: _____

☐ Tests; Diagnosic, Staging, or Follow-up (e.g. blood studies, radiologic studies)

| Test Name | Facility Name | Test Name | Facility Name |
|---|---|---|---|
| | | | |

☐ Treatment
Goal: (check one) ☐ Curative ☐ Palliative ☐ Concurrent chemotherapy

| Region to be treated | No. of Fields | Fields/Day | Total Dose | Dose/Day | No. Fractions |
|---|---|---|---|---|---|
| | | | | | |

☐ Consultants/Referrals
☐ Specialty _____  ☐ Specialty _____
Provider's Name _____  Provider's Name _____
Facility Name _____  Facility Name _____

☐ Hospitalization  Facility Name _____ Admit Date _____ Anticipated LOS _____
☐ Other

**CLINICAL PLAN RATIONALE (Briefly indicate reason for Clinical Plan)**
☐ Clinical Plan Diagnosis  ☐ Second Opinion
☐ Disease Progression  ☐ Abnormal Lab Values (attatched)
☐ Complications Secondary to Therapy  ☐ Other; _____

STEP 1 — COMPLETE CLINICAL PLAN FORM
STEP 2 — FAX FORM AND ALL SUPPORTING DOCUMENTATION TO: _____

* See reverse for data items to be included with initial Clinical Plan.

(a)

**Figure 5.3** Plan of care request forms: (a) radiation oncology and (b) medical oncology.

FOR SALICKNET *USE ONLY*
- ❏ *Requested Received* _____ _____
  - *Time* _____ *Date*
- ❏ *Product #* _____
- ❏ *Guideline Name* _____
- ❏ *Guideline Compliance?:* ❏ *Yes* ❏ *No* ❏ *N/A*
- ❏ *Date Entry by* _____ *(Initial/Date)*

# SAMPLE FORM

## MEDICAL ONCOLOGY
### CLINICAL PLAN

**Phase of Care**
**(Check all that apply)**
- ❏ Diagnosis
- ❏ Staging
- ❏ Therapy
- ❏ Follow-up

**Urgency (check one)**
- ❏ Routine
- ❏ **STAT**

### GENERAL INFORMATION

Member ID# _____  Member Name _____
_____ Last _____ First _____ Middle

Physician Name _____  Diagnosis _____  Stage _____

### CLINICAL PLAN (Complete all areas that apply)   Anticipated Start Date: _____

❏ **Tests; Diagnosic, Staging, or Follow-up** (e.g. blood studies, radiologic studies)

| Test Name | Facility Name | Test Name | Facility Name |
|---|---|---|---|
| | | | |
| | | | |

❏ **Treatment Therapy** Ht _____ Wt _____ BSA _____ Re-evaluation after _____ #courses  ❏ Concurrent radiation therapy

Drug Name, Dose (m²and actual), and Route    Frequency/Number of Courses

❏ **Consults/Referrals**

❏ Specialty _____     ❏ Specialty _____
Provider's Name _____     Provider's Name _____
Facility Name _____     Facility Name _____

❏ **Hospitalization**  Facility Name _____  Admit Date _____  Anticipated LOS _____

❏ **Other**

### CLINICAL PLAN RATIONALE (Briefly indicate reason for Clinical Plan)

- ❏ Clinical Plan Diagnosis
- ❏ Document Clinical Response
- ❏ Disease Progression
- ❏ Complications Secondary to Therapy
- ❏ Second Opinion
- ❏ Abnormal Lab Values (attached)
- ❏ Other; _____
  _____
  _____

*AUTHORIZATIONS*   Clinical Plan Approved?  ❏ *Completely*  ❏ *Partially (see comments)*  ❏ *No (see comments)*

*Physician Name* _____ *Auth#* _____ *Exp Date* _____

*Facility Name* _____ *Auth#* _____ *LOS* _____ *Exp Date* _____

*Authorization decision by* _____ *Title* _____ *Date* _____

*COMMENTS:*

**STEP 1**
COMPLETE CLINICAL
PLAN FORM

**STEP 2**
FAX FORM AND ALL
SUPPORTING
DOCUMENTATION TO: _____

\* See reverse for data items to be included with initial Clinical Plan.

(b)

**Figure 5.3** contd

(1) elective admissions for chemotherapy that could be administered safely in appropriate outpatient facilities or (2) treatment-related toxicity that may be mitigated by identifying cases at risk and intervening early with preventive measures.

An analysis over a 6-month period of elective chemotherapy admissions revealed that about 30% could have been safely performed in the outpatient setting without compromising quality of care.

In fact, it could be argued that quality of care would be improved by avoiding the immobilisation and exposure to infection that may occur with hospitalisation. The reasons for admission were discovered to be lack of outpatient resources within the physician's office, or lack of physician's familiarity with infusion devices such as intravenous catheters and pumps, which could safely be used in the outpatient setting. The lengthy experience with outpatient therapy within the SHC Cancer Centers made this a particularly simple problem to address. Most significant was that other physicians within the same network were providing the same therapy in the outpatient setting. The response to this finding was education of the admitting physicians and their nursing staff.

Admission for treatment-related toxicity was also analysed. Over a 6-month period, 47 admissions for toxicity were evaluated within one health plan, the causes being fever, sepsis, dehydration and diarrhoea (Table 5.2).

**Table 5.2** Admissions for treatment-related toxicity

| No. of admissions | Diagnosis | Total days | Average LOS |
|---|---|---|---|
| 13 | Fever | 54 | 4 |
| 20 | Sepsis | 144 | 7 |
| 13 | Dehydration | 65 | 5 |
| 1 | Diarrhoea | 8 | 8 |
| **47** | | **271** | **6** |

LOS, length of stay.

In most cases, the patients were receiving chemotherapy known to cause profound neutropenia or gastrointestinal toxicity, therefore allowing prediction of likelihood of toxicity. A process was developed for simple telephone follow-up by SalickNet case managers after high-risk chemotherapy, and the referral to the treating physicians for hydration or growth factor support to prevent admissions for advanced toxicity.

## Adequate diagnosis and staging – avoiding unnecessary surgery

An example of this aspect of care is therapy for early stage prostate cancer. Both surgery and radiotherapy are considered curative for early stage prostate cancer. Yet, not all patients are adequately staged to confirm their eligibility for such therapy and, once staged, not all patients are offered radiotherapy as an alternative to surgery.

The SalickNet approach was to institute two major guidelines for any patient for whom surgery was requested. First, a preoperative bone scan was required for any patient with a prostate-specific antigen (PSA) level > 10. This was based on data in the medical literature indicating that as many as 10% of such patients may be found to have metastatic disease, rendering surgery inappropriate. Within the first 6 months of applying this guideline, 20% of planned prostatectomy patients were found to have stage IV disease, and surgery was aborted. The second guideline was to insist that a radiotherapy consultation be offered to all patients intended for surgery, to allow them the option to consider radiotherapy, if they wished to avoid surgery. Similar programmes were instituted for the preoperative staging of lung cancer and colorectal cancer.

## Ensuring a multidisciplinary approach to care

All patients with diagnoses for which combined modality therapy was considered the standard of care – stage III breast cancer, stage III lung cancer, stage III rectal cancer, stage III laryngeal cancer, etc. – were identified, and surgery would not be approved until consultation with medical and radiation oncology specialists was offered, and arranged by SalickNet. In many cases, surgery was preceded by radiotherapy and/or chemotherapy, offering the potential for downstaging of tumours, and better likelihood of long-term benefit.

## Ensuring appropriate use of supportive medications

Growth factors to elevate white blood cell counts after chemotherapy are widely used by US oncologists. As a result of the significant cost of these agents, and the potential for over-utilisation, the American Society of Clinical Oncology (ASCO) issued guidelines for their use in 1994, with an update in 1996. As these guidelines were voluntary, they had little impact on physician practices. Within the HMO system managed by SalickNet, significant overuse of these factors was observed. The action taken was to apply the ASCO guidelines to the oncology network, and to provide education regarding the appropriate use of these agents. All requests for use of these agents were required to conform to ASCO guidelines. The result was a striking reduction in use of these agents, without a concomitant increase in toxicity of therapy or other negative consequences. Most importantly, no increase in admission for neutropenic fever was noted (Figure 5.4).

## Effect of SalickNet disease management of cancer in a managed care system

Over 5 years of operation, SalickNet achieved a variety of goals which improved quality of care while accomplishing cost reduction for the health plans involved. In the area of quality of care, SalickNet provided co-ordination of complex care plans in a fragmented system. Programmes such as pain management and toxicity

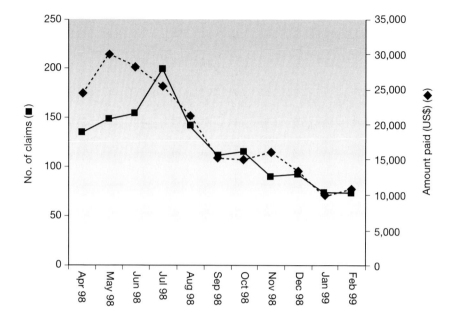

**Figure 5.4** Use of growth factors: trend for granulocyte colony-stimulating factor (G-CSF) and granulocyte–macrophage CSF (GM-CSF).

management were instituted. In certain disease types, significant improvements were documented. In breast cancer, late diagnosis was detected and acted on by improving screening, choice between lumpectomy with radiation vs mastectomy was routinely offered, and use of adjuvant therapy for curable stages was standardised. Adjuvant therapy was also standardised for curable stages of colorectal cancer. In prostate cancer, education regarding the proper use of staging studies led to the avoidance of unnecessary (and potentially harmful) surgery in a significant number of patients.

Direct costs were reduced by the reduction of hospitalisations for febrile neutropenia and for elective chemotherapy. Costs were reduced by decreasing unnecessary utilisation of growth factors, as well as unnecessary surgery. The indirect costs, which were avoided by improving the overall quality of care and accuracy of diagnosis, are difficult to quantify, but are likely to be substantial.

## Challenges to the success of oncology disease management in managed care

SalickNet was developed as a subsidiary of SHC, which would offer disease management services to managed care organisations on a contractual basis. As such, methods for assessing the success of disease management were required. For most managed care organisations, the goals of acquiring disease management services are cost reduction and improvements in quality of care. For cost reduction to be achieved in the area of cancer care, some determination of cancer-related costs before disease management was required. In the two major contracts entered into by SalickNet, pre-existing cancer costs could not be accurately determined based on existing health plan databases, as a result of the fragmented nature of cancer care. Therefore, no baseline existed against which to measure SalickNet performance, and the relative magnitude of short-term cost reduction was difficult to determine. Long-term cost reduction, which might occur with improving quality of care, such as improved screening and early diagnosis, could not be estimated over the period of time in which SalickNet operated.

The nature of healthcare coverage in the USA, including managed care, is such that individuals may change their coverage quite frequently, as employers change health plans. The managed care industry therefore often consider short-term goals, such as cost reduction, to take precedence over long-term goals that may be irrelevant to a patient population, which may leave their system within 2–5 years. Although the clinical and non-fiscal outcomes of disease management may have important relevance to public health, the short-term goals of the for-profit managed care industry raise doubts as to the utility of disease management in their unique market. For this reason, SHC is no longer involved in cancer disease management within the managed care system.

## SHC and oncology disease management – looking forward

SHC continues to manage comprehensive cancer centres throughout the USA, and is expanding into additional centres. The model of comprehensive cancer care and disease management is the basis of the design and operation of these cancer centres, and is easily applied to new locations and healthcare systems. The experience of managing cancer care within large managed care systems has established the ability of the cancer disease management approach to improve quality of care successfully while reducing costs when appropriate. This approach may have limited appeal for the US system of managed health care as currently configured. However, it is clearly of benefit to healthcare systems in which long-term public health goals are combined with the need to utilise limited healthcare resources efficiently. As a result, in addition to the US cancer centre network, SHC is also exploring the potential application of oncology disease management outside the USA, where nationally funded healthcare systems may derive the greatest benefit from this approach.

*References*

*Los Angeles Times* (2000). The California nightmare. *Los Angeles Times* 20 Nov

Mighion K, Gesme D, Rifkin M, Bennet C (1999). Growth of oncology physician practice management companies. *Cancer Investigation* **17**, 362–370

Reynolds S (1999). Commercial managed care. *Cancer Investigation* **17**, 434–440

Chapter 6

# Adaptable networks: perspectives from a business context

*Jane M Gillies and Ian P McCarthy*

## Introduction

In the past few years, the idea of networks has been enthusiastically taken up in planning and policy making. Increasingly, what is commonly termed a 'network approach' is regarded as a desirable way forward in economic development, in public services provision and especially in the health service. From a policy level perspective, the NHS is committed to the development of network structures in a number of different areas of care and to the continued provision of care in such network form. Although some initiatives are already well under way, especially in cancer care – and the Scottish experience is useful in this sense – there is still a wide-ranging debate within the NHS about what constitutes a network, where the model came from and why it is being adopted.

This chapter seeks to address these questions by presenting a network model and a view of network behaviours drawn from the business context. The model is based on research into flexible, adaptable, self-organising networks in business. Such industrial networks, as they are known, have been identified in a number of industries that are predominantly fast-paced, highly innovative and highly unpredictable sectors, such as the fashion garment industry, biotechnology and information technology (IT). The chapter starts with a review of network definitions and focuses on the industrial network model. An example of this model operating successfully is described in the case of the Italian district networks. Focusing on the business model, the environment and the rationales for behaviour in the network are examined, and the key features characterising this form are identified. On the basis of these, the ability of the network to be adaptable is explained. The focus widens to examine the advantages and disadvantages of networks and to identify specifically what networks are good for. This leads naturally to the question of why an organisation would seek to move to a network structure. From this basis, the chapter focuses on the implications of transferring and applying this model to a health service context.

The aim in presenting the model does not imply that this is what would constitute a successful network within the health service; rather it helps address the key question of what would be a successful network form for the NHS.

## What is a network?

As with many words, the term 'network' has lost precision, and its meaning has altered over the years. The *New Shorter Oxford English Dictionary* makes reference to its original use to denote the way in which a particular fabric or work had been made – 'work in which threads, wires, etc., are crossed or interlaced in the fashion of a net'. *Roget's Thesaurus* offers a number of synonyms: 'plexus, mesh, reticle, chain, group interconnection.' Today the word has come to be used in a wide range of contexts to express interconnectedness of different kinds. The most suitable definition for the present purpose is 'a chain or system of interconnected or intercommunicating immaterial things, points or people' from the *New Shorter Oxford English Dictionary*. The usage of the word is now widespread in numerous contexts from business and management to IT, sociology, economics and geography. In each case definitions become more precise as they are used to describe specific systems, for example, a social network is described as a set of nodes (e.g. people, organisations), linked by a set of social relationships (e.g. friendship, transfer of funds, overlapping membership) of a specific type.

Axelsson and Easton (1992), in the introduction to their edited volume on industrial networks, define them as follows:

> . . . in the case of industrial networks as opposed to say social, communication or electrical networks, the entities are actors involved in the economic processes which convert resources to finished goods and services for consumption by end users whether they be individuals or organisations. Thus the links between actors are usually defined in terms of economic exchanges which are themselves conducted within the framework of an enduring relationship. The existence of such relationships are the raison d'être for industrial networks

The flexibility and universality of the term are an indication that a network is not necessarily a rigidly defined entity that can be concisely defined and captured. In recognition of this, network theorists talk rather of a network perspective, arguing that their organisations and behaviours are such 'elusive phenomena' that 'one could never hope for a definitive theory in the field. All that one could expect was the benefit of a perspective or a framework that could be used like a "walking stick" to support and navigate one's enquiry through the treacherous terrain of organisations' (Nohria & Eccles 1992). A network is therefore not necessarily a discrete and unchangeable entity which can easily be defined and given parameters. This feature of network forms may be a significant reason why they are so difficult to implement and set up. To underline this further, Easton (Axelsson & Easton 1992) offers a number of different views of networks as relationships, structure, process and position. These demonstrate that a network is as much about a way of behaving and being as about a particular organisational form.

Modern network theory is concerned with the study of particular forms and structures of socioeconomic organisation. In the last 15 years there has been a great increase of interest in forms of collaborative relationships between firms. Network forms have been hailed as the 'new competition' (Best 1990), the third organisational form (Powell 1990) and the organisational form for the 'information age' (Lipnack & Stamps 1994). Academically, networks have grown out of the critiques of early analyses of forms of economic organisation – in particular, Williamson's (1975) identification of the market or hierarchy spectrum. This linked organisational forms to the nature of economic transactions. Those transactions that involve uncertainty, recur frequently and require substantial investments were said to take place within hierarchically organised firms. Transactions that are straightforward, non-repetitive and not requiring investments were said to take place across a market interface. Any other form of economic organisation was said to be a hybrid form lying somewhere in between that spectrum. This analysis has been most influential in shaping economic and business thought since, but it also immediately gave rise to much criticism, not least because it ignored or did not acknowledge the embeddedness of economic action in a cultural and social context. Historians and sociologists contend that the market is not an amoral self-subsistent institution but a cultural and social construction. Network forms of economic organisation are now regarded as a third non-hybrid form, conferring substantial economic advantages, especially in environments that are uncertain, unpredictable and fast changing.

If the academic domain has recognised the importance of networks, this has been complemented by a great increase in the numbers of types of between-firm collaboration undertaken. This is a reflection of changing perceptions and a growing recognition of the benefits of networks.

Traditional models of the value chain picture it as a set of fixed relationships between specialists arranged in rigid series as product or value passes through (Figure 6.1). This was thought to be as true for automotive manufacture as for insurance service delivery. In this view, communication between nodes or functions was not considered necessary, product differentiation and customisation were limited, and the customer was the end node, standing outside the transformation process. The network perspective cuts across this reductionist, rationalist view, to one where populations of different experts exist in an overall community, and come together with the customer to meet specific needs. Figure 6.2 highlights the view that, in a network, only some of the nodes or actors come together each time. In this view, communication between nodes is vital for the achievement of the objectives, customisation and product differentiation are drivers for the system, and the customer is a partner in the process.

Comparing the two figures, it is clear how different these two views are, to the extent that they do not a replace each other in any way. Nor, however, are they mutually exclusive. Indeed, it is entirely possible to think of what takes place within a network as being represented by both images at different levels of abstraction and analysis. While one is functional and objectified, the other represents relationships within an embedded context. Even Figure 6.2 is itself a stylised and static representation

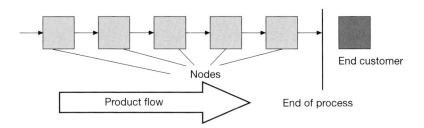

**Figure 6.1** Traditional value chain conceptualisation.

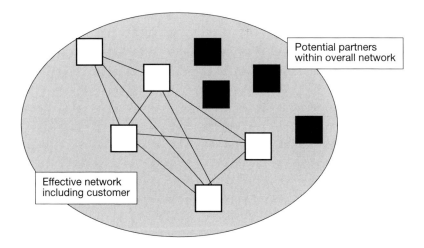

**Figure 6.2** Conceptualisation of network interactions.

of a network of relationships. A two-dimensional schematic cannot hope to capture the dynamic nature of such interactions, but here it serves to provide a contrast to relationships in Figure 6.1.

Network research has enabled the identification and differentiation of different types and categories of network, the 'totality of relationships among firms engaged in production, distribution and the use of goods and services in what might be described as an industrial system' (Axelsson & Easton 1992, p 3). It is not surprising therefore that the forms and types identified are diverse and ever changing. Researchers have struggled to bring order to this area, as more and more economic relationships are being recognised as taking place within the context of some form of network. In addition, adding to the confusion, the current popularity of the network concept has led to its appearance and use in a far greater number of instances, some of them at odds with each other.

Nohria and Eccles (1992) identify three levels at which networks occur: the entrepreneurial network firm, small firm networks such as those found in several industrial districts of Italy, and network-like economies such as those found in Japan, Korea and Taiwan. Perrow goes further still to provide a global map of the huge range of network forms (Figure 6.3), showing that some are more common in the USA, whereas others are found more frequently in Europe and the Far East. Perrow's start point is the 'Integrated Firm' model, which 'buys out as many of its competitors as it can and integrates backward and forward to control as much as it can of the throughput from raw materials to final consumer' (Perrow, cited in Nohria & Eccles 1992, p 445). In Perrow's description, we can recognise the Fordist model of vertical integration. He notes that, in the USA, there has been a move away from the integrated firm, towards more devolved structures, and provides three arguments for the move away:

1. Flexible production: smaller groupings of co-operating firms are better able to respond to the flexible production needs of today's markets.
2. Capitalist failure: the shedding of risk by the larger companies through subcontracting out to smaller independent units.
3. Organisational failure: through the supposed growth of large firms beyond a sustainable size.

Other classifications of network forms of business organisation begin from different perspectives. Easton and Araujo (cited in Axelsson & Easton 1992) offer a classification based on the presence of economic dimensions of exchange. They examine, in turn, the implications for relationships that do or do not involve economic exchange and where actors are directly and indirectly connected. They couple their classification to discussions of conflict and competition as well as co-operation between actors who find themselves vertically or horizontally linked in the value chain, and explore the extent to which network forms challenge or concur with traditional analyses of value chain relationships.

Based on these simple distinctions they build a taxonomy of forms of between-competitor co-operation, shown in Figure 6.4 (Axelsson & Easton 1992, p 77). The more formal arrangements are becoming increasingly familiar, and are 'overt, planned and managed', whereas the more informal relationships are 'much more likely to be individual, random and unplanned' (Easton & Araujo, cited in Axelsson & Easton 1992).

The formal/informal distinction is a useful and sensible one. Research suggests that this is one of the keys, if not in fact the most important factor, in determining the nature of between-firm relationships, the form of the network, the kinds of transactions taking place within it and their resultant histories. Certainly, the degree to which network actors feel that their relationships and interactions are subject to their own

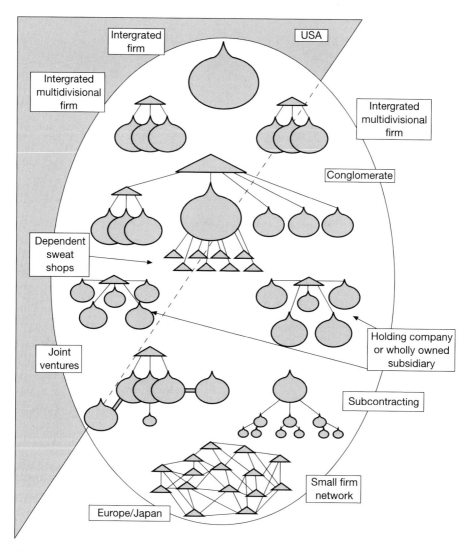

**Figure 6.3** Perrow's table of other forms of economic organisation (Perrow, cited in Nohria & Eccles 1992, p 447).

free will or are formally set out and predetermined will dictate the form of these relationships. In the pursuit of individual aims and objectives, each actor must make the choice about whether to pursue them on a solitary, opportunistic basis or to seek to do so in collaboration with others. For each, this is essentially a decision about whether a solitary or a collaborative approach will yield the best results. The outcomes of the decisions made are embodied in what we perceive as social relations, the structure of communication systems, hierarchies and behavioural norms.

Direct                     Indirect

|                                | Direct | Indirect |
|--------------------------------|:------:|:--------:|
| Involving economic exchange    |   1    |    2     |
| Not involving economic exchange |   3    |    4     |

**Figure 6.4**  Classification of types of network relationship (Axelsson & Easton 1992).

## The Italian district networks – a success story

Industrial networks have been identified and studied as dynamic business organisational forms in a number of industries. Perhaps the best known, and certainly the earliest to be identified (Marshall 1890), are the networks found in certain areas of central and northern Italy. The 'Third Italy', as this area has come to be known, is a roughly triangular region comprising a string of industrial districts (IDs) stretching from Venice in the north to Ancona in the south and centred on Bologna and Florence (Becattini 1990). Historically, this was the epicentre of the medieval Italian merchant city states that financed the birth of the European Renaissance. These deep roots generated a social environment that fostered craftsmanship, commercial *nouse* and civilised competition alongside expedient co-operation. In the period after World War II, these areas have increasingly become centres for innovation and technologically sophisticated production. IDs are estimated to account for 45% of manufacturing employment in Italy, 40% of exports and 20% of gross national product (GNP) (Biggiero 1999). Their commercial success is complemented by high employment records, high productivity, high incomes and good labour relations. These benefits are attributed to the development of the unique identity and internal organisation of the IDs.

For the greater part of the twentieth century the Italian IDs defied accepted management wisdom which, as discussed above, did not recognise the importance of networks. A challenge to Fordism, they pre-date it, having initially been identified by Marshall in 1890. Since then, they have attracted increasing attention, and especially so in the past 20 years. The reason for this attention lies in their commercial success, which has endured since Marshall's first description. The districts have weathered the twentieth century storms. Through times of poverty, increasing industrialisation, two world wars, mass production, Far Eastern competition and globalisation, they have continued to be successful. The source of their success is regarded as being the result of their **adaptability** and their resulting ability to co-evolve with their external environment. This adaptability may be regarded as taking two forms.

## Microadaptability

In the shorter term, and on an individual basis, the actors in the ID are able to adapt to changing market requirements. This ability has been labelled flexible specialisation and derives from a coupling of individual specialisation with a tradition of craftsmanship.

## Macroadaptability

In the mid to long term, and on a district basis, the ID is able to adapt to changing external environment conditions. Through this century, IDs have changed from agriculture-based artisan production, to the adoption of up-to-date technology, and now to an increased emphasis on knowledge about intensive aspects of value such as service and design.

Industrial districts have been defined by Becattini (1990) as spatially and culturally identifiable areas in which both employers and employees live and work. Ideally they comprise numerous small firms engaged in activities related to a single industrial category. Moreover, they are located within a clearly identifiable community in terms of geography, history and culture. Cultural influences produce an atmosphere of co-operation and trust in which economic action is regulated by a series of implicit and explicit rules governed by social conventions and by public and private organisations (Lazerson & Lorenzoni 1998). Coro and Grandinetti (1999, p 117) identify three key characteristics of IDs:

1. A large number of small and medium-sized firms that are specialised both horizontally and vertically.
2. Wide-ranging integrated competencies that are rooted in a particular geographical area and that shape a specific unified local labour market.
3. A relational system that allows production to be co-ordinated efficiently inside a technical cluster through both competition and co-operation assets.

Where an industrial network is a set of relationships between actors engaged in a shared industrial activity, IDs are comprised of networks of such actors bounded by geographical locatedness. Several such networks may be linked in the same ID. Biggiero (1999) uses the term 'hypernetwork', where he distinguishes between three nested levels of the term network:

1. Intra-organisational: network between actors in one organisation.
2. Inter-organisational: network of relationships within which an organisation exists.

3. Hypernetwork: networks of firm networks, an accumulation of the level above.

In this sense, hypernetworks are networks of networks, and IDs are regional hypernetworks, i.e. 'networks of inter-organisational (institutional and economic) networks in a defined area' (Biggiero 1999, p 74).

The geographical boundedness of the ID has been an important aspect of its identity. It is thought that the proximity of the network actors has enabled the development of strong relationships and trust formation, essential to collaboration. Increasingly, however, Lazerson and Lorenzoni (1998) find that outsourcing is taking place, either in sourcing supplies or in subcontracting. They believe that this begins to challenge the view that IDs are of necessity geographically fixed. Information technology has also contributed to this trend. At the same time, however, they also comment that it is the low value-added and intermediate phases of production that are being subcontracted, whereas the essential, high value-added activities of design, final inspection, marketing and distribution remain concentrated within the district (Lazerson & Lorenzoni 1998). It remains to be seen whether these trends herald an end to the success of IDs. Biggiero (1999, p 81) points out that, although geographical boundaries may be dissolving, 'aspects of social psychology suggest that face-to-face relationships and spatial proximity are to remain highly important for human communication and for trust formation in particular'.

IDs are overwhelmingly composed of small enterprises. Over 50% of the workforce in the districts are employed by companies with fewer than 20 employees (Becattini 1990). Indeed, Best (1990) makes the point that, although in the 1970s and 1980s Italy had the fastest growth rate of the four biggest European economies (and surpassed the UK and France to become the fourth largest capitalist economy), this growth rate was not associated with a shift from small to large companies. This is the direct antithesis of industrialisation trends in other countries. This is not to say that there are no larger companies, but rather it is the case that small enterprises are in the majority.

A key success factor of the IDs is what has been called flexible specialisation. In manufacturing terms this reflects the juxtaposition of specialisation and multi-skilling in a narrow area of production that characterises the 'craftsman' approach. Sabel (1986) distinguishes between the large firm variant and the small firm variant. Although the former is concerned with issues internal to the firm, the latter is where flexible specialisation results from the clustering of small firms and a strong between-firm division of labour. Individual action and specialisation in this context are meaningless and futile; they must be linked closely within a network of specialisations along the whole of the value chain. For this reason close relationships between firms are the key to flexible specialisation. Moreover, success depends on a mutually accepted and respected division of labour which maximises firm-specific competencies. Effectively this creates interdependencies between actors which allow them to be collectively flexible and responsive, providing a 'strategic leverage in accomplishing and maintaining a sustainable competitive advantage' (Lipparini & Sobrero 1994, p 127). It also creates the opportunity for roles that transcend the simple functional breakdown of production activities. The pressures of co-ordination give rise to **agency** roles, concerned with the collection and distribution of information, knowledge, plans and strategy (Sabel 1986).

Relationships between firms are considered crucial in enabling this unique division of labour to take place. For some the relational capability of the individual firm is the one key factor to its successful existence in this milieu. Research indicates that this capability encompasses the ability of the firm to form mutually satisfying relationships with others, the experience of such relationships built up over time, the importance given to them, the numbers of such relationships engaged in and the success rate. Biggiero presents this in the form of a number of positive feedback processes, shown in Figure 6.5. The key to relationships of this nature is the development of trust, mutual respect and commitments. In IDs these relationships are embedded and take place within a social milieu that fosters them and which in turn is borne out of them. According to Sabel (1986) this is a matter of a particular way of life. Trust, reciprocity, the importance of reputation and the development of long-term relationships all contribute to this milieu. This can be contrasted with modern network building attempts, where trust building is regarded as an essential functional step, but it is de-coupled from the social context where it develops in truth. The understanding that relationships are long term involves an acceptance of long-term commitment, wherein memory and reputation begin to play a key role. The interactions take place in a geographically, socially and culturally bounded environment. Behaviours and their outcomes are noted by the others who also inhabit this environment. In turn, this increases or decreases the social capital of the participants, and influences the decision of others about whether to engage in future interactions with them.

Co-operation and competition in the ID are coexistent and co-dependent. As well as co-operation between actors vertically aligned in the value chain, there is also

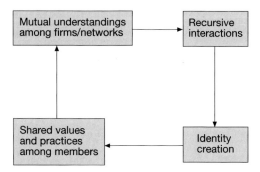

**Figure 6.5** Positive feedback processes in hypernetwork identity (Biggiero 1999, p 79).

co-operation between actors horizontally aligned, traditionally seen as competitors. Yet, this is a form of co-operation which, far from stifling competition, in fact aids it. Competitiveness thus 'emerges as a network-embedded capacity' (Lipparini & Sobrero 1994, p 127), which is actualised through the co-ordination of labour. The presence of co-operation among competitors does not mean that competition among them is eliminated, and this enables better option search, creativity and innovation, driven by a striving for individual success. All this adds up to a delicate balance between co-operation and competition. In the literature rationales are provided as to why firms would co-operate, based on a mix of historical, social, cultural, economic and other reasons (Becattini 1990; Best 1990). This work in turn has given rise to a counter-literature which illustrates where co-operation does not work and fierce competition abounds. However, this is to place all the emphasis on a non-dynamic, deterministic understanding of the balance between co-operation and competition. At an underlying level, actors make their choice based on their own evaluations of the benefits or penalties of each, across a number of dimensions – social and economic. In some environments, these social dimensions carry a higher cost, but in others they do not. In the long run, the consequences of the aggregate choices made are evident. The important thing is, however, that the balance is something that is context specific and based on the totality of the subjective judgements made. Thus, we can find instances where firms choose to co-operate or to compete, even if ultimately this carries too high an economic cost, as shown by the cases of the Leicestershire hosiery industry and that of the Bolognese silk industry described by Lazerson and Lorenzoni (1999). In the research, this shows that economic failure results, with the collapse of an economic activity in an area. As many of the UK's former industrial areas show, this also heralds the collapse of the social environment.

The division and co-ordination of labour, co-operation, trust and the accompanying social milieu enable the sharing of knowledge and the development of further knowledge in common. For the individual actors, this means focusing on what they do best, while acquiring inputs and knowledge about other activities in the chain of value from collaborators. In their empirical study of IDs, Lipparini and Sobrero (1994, p 129) found that 'relying on external sources, enables firms to introduce new products that better fit customers' requirements. All the firms described at length the advantages of having an efficient set of collaborative suppliers'. Thus each actor is able to bring to bear his or her expertise and knowledge in the joint collaborative activity shared with other actors. Out of this co-ordination comes knowledge fission, a shared knowledge and experience, between the actors involved, about that particular experience and each other. Farinelli (1996) calls this the tacit knowledge of the IDs, and says that often it is specific to that cluster of enterprises and is usually accumulated over a lengthy historical period.

IDs cannot simply be understood as production mechanisms; they are complex multidimensional systems – economic, social, cognitive, cultural and symbolic. They have within them the ability to co-evolve with their external environment. The evidence according to Lazerson (1988, p 331) 'seems to indicate that small firm expansion depends on a particular social and political order'. The internal organisation of the networks is made possible through the presence of reinforcing external organisations and institutions, what has come to be known as the D factor. The role of political traditions and institutions, such as the trade unions and the Italian communist party, have been shown to have exercised a decisive influence over the way in which the networks have developed. Becattini (1990, p 154) states that a dimension of political activity has been the 'creation of a full system of formal and informal social institutions acting as *"socialising agencies"* that bind people together, at work, at home and in leisure time'. Local institutions play an important role in ensuring harmony between public and private values, and in providing support, sources of knowledge and expertise in the ID.

A most significant feature of Italian industrial networks is the recognition of the important role of agency and the importance of agents – perhaps most famously in the district of Prato, where they are known locally as *impannatori*. These are organisations and individuals who undertake the development and marketing of the product lines. That states their role in bald terms. The work of the *impannatori* is concerned with knowledge at a deeper level than a purely functional breakdown of the task can capture. To understand this more, it is necessary to recognise the importance of exploration and knowledge search in the industrial districts. In all the interviews conducted as part of this study, and in further interviews conducted within other districts, one activity was emphasised above all – that of constantly seeking new information about the market, competitors and new developments. In Prato, this role is taken on predominantly by the *impannatori*. They seek to learn about new markets, new products, technologies and sources, even when times are good. They also seek to know about the capabilities and nature, on an on-going basis, of the other organisations in the value chain within the district, and further afield. This constant search for new information and knowledge is directly put to use in the functional role of the *impannatori*, in developing and marketing product lines. Their skills lie in selecting what will be produced, bringing together other firms to produce this and finally marketing it. As a result, the role of the *impannatori* is that of *knowledge agents*. They perform the knowledge management tasks that are increasingly recognised as vital to success. As a result, the industry is constantly updated and well informed about current developments, and is able to offer an up-to-date response. As a result of the *impannatori*, the industry in the district has become more automated and stayed at the forefront of technological developments and utilisation. This is assisted by the presence of several textile machinery manufacturers in the area.

This brief review of the Italian district networks gives some idea of their nature and operation. From this body of work and research in this area, it is possible to draw out key features and characteristics of a successful network. Indeed a list of this kind is presented below. One important caveat must be made at this point, however, which is that the Italian networks did not happen yesterday or indeed in the last decade. They are the product of a way of life and a social environment that has been in place or developing for some time. Is it possible to pick out the key features and to attempt to re-create such an environment? It is advisable to proceed with caution in doing so.

## A network model

The following sections of this chapter introduce a model that allows the different configurations and behaviours of an industrial network to be understood. It focuses on several characteristics, including: the external environment; flexibility and adaptability; resources and knowledge; values; power; and self-organisation.

### The network environment

The network environment is socially a familiar one. Interactions and exchanges of a particular kind take place, but they do so on terms that are to a great extent familiar to us all from our personal experience. The network in this sense does not have a distinct boundary any more than our personal networks of contacts have any specific boundary. Instead, it is characterised by a permeable, flexible boundary, which stretches and contracts dynamically. This is reflected in the definition of the network model presented here, as a self-organised co-ordination of value chain activities among actors, some of them firms, some of them teams or individuals. The network is based on a trust-based potentiality for collaboration among individuals, some of them competitors, who share knowledge and information. It is characterised by being flexible and adaptable in response to the environment that it inhabits and co-evolving with it.

On the basis of this, the key features of a network have been identified (Gillies 2000) as being the following.

### *Flexibility and adaptability*

From a number of different perspectives, networks are regarded as offering advantages over other forms of economic organisation. Most significantly, in the management literature, they are recognised as offering flexibility and agility of response at a time when markets overall are becoming more unpredictable, more unstable, both bigger and smaller, and more demanding. Mass customisation and globalisation are two trends that are seen to be changing the competitive landscape. Both require increased responsiveness across all sectors. Both are also pushing competition to take place on the basis of differentiation rather than on price, as has been more the case in the past. The implications are for an increased emphasis and reliance on the knowledge component of product design and delivery. Across these domains – differentiation, knowledge-based responses, responsiveness – networks are recognised as having advantages over more cumbersome larger organisations that are slow to turn around and respond. They also have advantages over the individual firm competing alone in the market, because it has to rely entirely on its own efforts for everything, and hence cannot hope to cover all alternatives and possibilities. Networks allow small, flexible units to gain access to a much wider body of knowledge about market needs, know-how, etc. and to harness this flexibility in response. They are able to adapt more rapidly to market needs as a result, and thus to be more competitively successful in the given market conditions. Networks are therefore able to deliver and be successful in:

- fast-moving unpredictable environments
- customised, heterogeneous products/services
- innovative ways.

### Sharing resources and knowledge

The particular co-ordination of work that networks allow enables individual units such as firms to gain access to previously unattainable sources of knowledge and resources through sharing. In particular, knowledge sharing and co-creation are regarded as key competitive advantages of networks. This results in part from the changing nature of markets today, where competition is increasingly based on differentiation and flexibility. This leads inevitably to a focus on design, innovation and knowledge-based added value. Networks confer an increased ability for small flexible enterprises to access a greater body of knowledge in a way that would otherwise be impossible. Successful relationships and progress in networks depend on the interactions between companies taking the form of knowledge exchange and co-creation. Knowledge is not limited to technical, product knowledge; it is also knowledge of each other. One of the first things that begins to grow in a network, before any profit-generating collaboration has taken place, is shared knowledge of each other by the participating actors or organisations. Such knowledge is directly related to the form of relationship that exists between network actors.

### A balance between collaboration and competition

The effective network is to be found inhabiting the middle ground somewhere between purely competitive and purely co-operative behaviour, as shown in Figure 6.6. It is readily understandable why competitive behaviour does not lead to effective network behaviours, but what is equally important is that purely co-operative or collaborative behaviour is also detrimental, leading to insularity, tunnel vision and a clique mentality, all of which weaken the ability to understand and respond to external conditions. The network is effective because it is open just enough to be affected by new inputs and competitors, but not enough to make life too threatening and competitive for its participants. It is effectively a trade-off between the two forces of competition and collaboration.

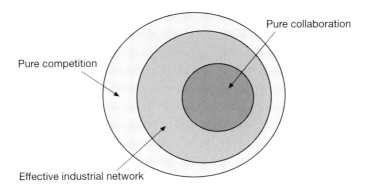

**Figure 6.6** Location of effective network behaviours.

## Predicated on the importance of relationships

Rationalist analysis may lead to the conclusion that networks are based on altruistic decisions made by individual network actors. These underlying decisions drive initial behaviour, but their outcome results in patterns of behaviour that become the raison d'être of the network: the relationships between the actors. In the network these relationships are based on trust and mutual understanding, and on the whole tend to be collaborative. The basis of network relationships is examined in greater detail below, but here it is important to stress the emphasis that is placed by network actors on the development of good trusting relationships among themselves.

## The sharing of common values

Within a network, relationships are crucial; they are the glue with the strength to make the network more or less successful. Effective collaboration is thus contingent on the development and existence of a set of commonly held perceptions and values between network actors and on the resulting development of long-term relationships. Such common cognitive structures build commitment and trust over the longer term. Within networks relationships between actors take place over a longer time horizon than is commonly assumed to be the case. The sharing of qualitative, tacit knowledge, such as know-how, a particular approach to production or design or a style of doing business, can take place only where there is an understanding of longer-term commitment, and a common obligation and interests. In turn this builds trust and confidence to engage in further exchange and sharing. In Grabher's (1993) words, 'network forms of exchange entail indefinite, sequential transactions within the context of a general pattern of reciprocity', where reciprocity is defined as 'actions that are contingent on rewarding reactions from others and that cease when these expected reactions are not forthcoming' (Blau 1964). Reciprocity plays a central role but is a complex ambiguous term that is not simply the reciprocation of good turns – it also encompasses bad turns, as Axelrod (1984) points out.

The sociological and anthropological literature has concerned itself with questions of whether reciprocity implies equivalence of benefits, whether there is a relatively immediate assessment and return, and to what extent it confers indebtedness. Calculation, however, may well undermine the building of a relationship. Powell (1990) points out that the obligations to give, to receive and to return were not to be understood simply with respect to rational calculations, but fundamentally in terms of underlying cultural tenets that provide objects with their meaning and significance, and provide a basis for understanding the implications of their passage from one person to another. Reciprocity is only really meaningful in a social context, where as well as the participants there is also an audience to the transactions and exchanges, an audience that is made up of other potential participants. The undeniable social context of economic action, and the significance of reciprocity and ensuing levels of co-operation and trust have given rise to concepts of social capital (Alter & Hage 1993). Although exchange cost theorists would question the extent to which such cultural considerations play a role, undoubtedly networks involve relationships that are played out over many exchanges and interactions. In such a context, past experience will doubtless be part of the calculations of how to behave at present along with purely economic factors. This feature of networks is so important that it is worth a brief re-cap: network relationships are crucial, and are played out within long-term contexts, where the development of common understanding, common culture, language and habits reinforce the quality and depth of the relationship.

*Self-organisation, free will and power*

The co-ordination of work, reciprocity and the trust aspect of relationships within networks implies a degree of self-determination and free will on the part of the actors. In other words, the actors enter into these relationships to some extent through their own choice. Further, the relationships and the form that they take are to a great extent self-regulating. Order in networks is achieved through negotiated processes which evolve with the mutual adjustment of actors (Alter & Hage 1993). The co-ordination of work is to this extent self-organised, in the sense that it is not centrally planned and imposed. It would be wrong, however, to conceive of networks solely in terms of altruistic collaborations and friendships. Power may be defined as the possibility of imposing one's will on others, and authority as the means by which dominance is cloaked in legitimacy. Power imbalances are part of network life, as a functional element used in exploiting interdependencies. The power aspect of networks is subject to context. So, for example, while Burt (1992) sees power as a capacity conferred on the actor involved by the network that he or she is at the centre of, others set out a number of theory areas that view power as a function of the pursuit of the actor's self-interest. Nevertheless, although power balances within a network are a constantly shifting reality, this does not extend to the presence of a centralised power house within a network that has the ability to dictate action at all times.

The networks being described here are, to a great degree, self-organised and free from excessive external or internal centralisation of power.

### Interdependence and co-ordination of labour

The defining characteristics of a business network are collaboration and joint effort. These are the result of network actors accepting that they have common goals and objectives that cannot be reached separately. Mutual understanding of what can be done enables the network actors to co-ordinate their work together to meet these goals. As a result, a high degree of interdependence operates between network actors. This form of collaboration raises the issue of what the competitive unit is in this situation, and research in this area leads to the conclusion that it is by no means the traditional individual organisation. Within a network form of organisation, the effective competitive unit is the network as a whole, rather than the individual operational unit working together within it. In the collaborative process, shared goals and values are developed as well as the skill and ability to work together on a common task. Mutual understanding and common values are aspects of an environment of trust and common social values shared by network actors.

### Co-evolving with the environment

In seeking to understand the behaviour of networks, it is important to take into account both internal interactions and interactions with the external environment. The network is in this respect not a closed system, as Figure 6.1 would seem to indicate. This is a significant issue, for not only does the network as a whole interact with the external environment, but also internal interactions take place in the context of that environment. In other words, the network is an open dynamic system that is in co-evolution with its environment. Co-evolution goes beyond mere interaction; it takes place over the longer term and is not a one-off discrete event. The network produces responses to the environment. These responses trigger changes in the larger environment, which in turn lead to further responses from the network. The whole is prevented from spiralling into a positive feedback spiral by the existence of other, neighbouring systems that are diverse and also offer responses and co-evolve with the larger environment. Their diversity ensures that they do not have the same responses as each other, and hence the wider environment reacts differently each time. This pattern is evident in the behaviour of successful networks in industry which are constantly changing and shifting their composition and product/service in response to the needs of the environment. In turn these changes also change the needs of the environment itself.

## Network adaptability

The key features described above are important elements in seeking to understand networks, but they do not in themselves really present a coherent picture of how networks operate, change and adapt. Two important dynamics are at work within the effective network (Gillies 2000). The first concerns the individual choice that network actors make about whether to take part in the network or not, the second is about knowledge in the network.

Networks are composed of individual actors (organisations or people, or loose groups), who have made a decision about whether to collaborate with others or to act alone. The first dynamic is concerned with the basis on which this decision is made. In traditional analyses of behaviour and motivation, rational and selfish reasons are assumed to hold sway. However, that is to ignore the importance of reputation, friendship, trust and satisfaction from team effort – the particulars that relate to our wish to feel part of a social group, to feel recognition from others and love. It is possible that these are not taken into account because they are very difficult to evaluate in a quantitative manner. Moreover they are subjective measures, which bear different values for each person or social group. The decision to act and subsequent behaviour take place within the context of more than one potential interaction and in a wider social context. Behaviour is therefore public and visible for a great part and, as discussed above, reputation, reciprocity and memory are important elements of this overall dynamic. These values and reasons for behaviour are important, and constitute a 'mix' which varies between individuals. On the basis of this 'mix' we weigh each situation up and decide whether to collaborate or to act alone. This amounts to making a decision about whether to pursue our objectives alone or in collaboration with others. It must be noted here that the real question is not one of competition or collaboration, but of whether the objectives and the satisfaction of the 'mix' can best be achieved by either of these. It is useful to picture this as a set of scales with solitary action on one side and collaborative action on the other. The decision is based on the anticipated results of a course of action for each of the factors in the overall 'mix'. Faced with the choice between two courses of action, the network actor chooses that which has the most beneficial end-result, taking **all** factors into account. These may be summarised as follows:

- The degree to which a course of action will or will not satisfy the objectives of that actor.
- The potential of more than one interaction between the actors involved.
- Social context – witnessed by others.
- The importance of reputation and reciprocity in that context.
- The presence of build-up of social capital and its importance.
- The adherence and existence of formal and informal rules and modes of behaviour.

The second dynamic at work in the network is concerned with knowledge. At the heart of every network interaction and the development and production of a network response is the issue of knowledge and knowledge exchange. This again is not simply an issue of static or individual knowledge. There are many different kinds of knowledge, of which the conventional knowledge base appropriate to each level of education or training is only a small part. Moreover, knowledge is not static; it is constantly changing and being updated. In a network interaction, as two or more bodies of knowledge come together, important processes take place: knowledge is shared to a greater or lesser extent – with the significant risk of misinterpretation – and knowledge is also co-created, as each actor leaves the transaction having had their store of knowledge changed by it. In a dynamic, flexible network, the diversity of sources of knowledge generation and exchange are critical for the adaptability and innovativeness of the network. The following are of significance.

## Microdiversity and heterogeneity

In a network, actors are recognised as being different, even at the micro-level. These differences need not be significant, but they will serve to make each interaction unique. Heterogeneity implies greater differences, whereas microdiversity describes small differences between similar actors. The recognition and acceptance of both levels of difference between actors and variety overall in the network are important for its diversity and flexibility of response.

## The balance between collaboration and competition

As discussed above, the effective network takes place in the space between total collaboration and total competition. This balance serves to generate a dynamic tension in the network, driving out the complacency that can be the product of too much collaboration while offering some protection from the savagery of a totally competitive environment. In this dynamic tension, diversity and innovativeness flourish.

## Exploration and exploitation

Both of these are important and mutually dependent. Exploration is a precursor to exploitation of new knowledge, and without it there is nothing new to exploit. Exploitation, however, provides some stability and economies of scale, allowing resources to be created for the exploration process. There is a tendency in planning and designing organisations to view exploration as waste. Of necessity it is wasteful, because it is not always successful. Success rates for pharmaceutical exploration (R&D), for instance, are quoted at lower than 5%. This is a burden for any organisation to carry, but it must be accepted, for without it there can be no progression. Error making can be significant if it is treated as potential for learning. The major criticism of accountancy-based, cost-cutting, focused management planning is that it does not recognise the intrinsic value of this, seeking instead to optimise activity and performance in every single area. Unfortunately, this leads to an organisation where there is no 'slack', and which is then unable to deal with any deviations from the planned norm.

*Movement of knowledge in the network system*

Diversity of knowledge is of no use unless it is moving around the system well. This ability is governed by systems and levels of communication and how effective these are. Communication takes place along both formal and informal lines and can be hampered by both. Studies of successful networks in the central Italian districts distinguish and acknowledge the role of agents in this process – network actors whose role it is to gather and then distribute information and knowledge from both the network and its environment. In these networks, this role is seen as a crucial one and agents are at the centre of network interactions. Their skill in identifying what information is important and with whom to communicate is a significant contributing factor to the flexibility, adaptability and success of the network overall.

The functioning of the network is the product of the interplay between these two sets of dynamics, that of the drivers of individual choice and the knowledge factors. This interplay determines the degree of adaptability of the network, and results in a unique set of relationships between the network actors. Relationships develop as a result of freely made decisions about whether to collaborate or compete. On the basis of these decisions, knowledge and resources are shared and exchanged. Collaboration and interdependence result, and adaptability, flexibility and the other network advantages follow. At the start of the process, however, is the individual's decision about collaboration. It may be concluded that, to begin to develop a successful network, one must first place emphasis on the factors that drive that individual decision.

The network model presented is one that is constantly dynamic. Relationships change and develop continuously within it. As a result, a unique organisational form emerges that is suited to the very specific conditions of fast-paced, unpredictable markets. Indeed the research shows that this is where such networks are predominantly found. In these markets, there is a great need for wide-ranging exploration and experimentation in order to identify options and responses that the market will accept. The riskiness of such exploration is greatly diminished when it is shared among a number of collaborating actors. So there is a high incentive each time for the individual to collaborate. Accordingly, there is a great need for collaborative support structures, such as social capital and norms, importance to reputation and reciprocity, etc. These help to create trust and enable the sharing of knowledge. The network society thus comes into being. In such unpredictable, fast-moving environments networks make perfect sense, but they are not necessarily suited to more predictable, steadier situations, where market needs are known. Other forms and structures are better suited there. The important issue is to identify and recognise the nature of the environment and, on that basis, to decide whether a particular organisation structure is going to be suitable.

There is a significant degree of political will behind the drive towards networks, evident not only in the health sector but also in industry. The 1998 White Paper on

Competitiveness (Department of Trade and Industry 1988) stressed the importance of networks, clusters and collaboration 'The knowledge driven economy both facilitates and requires greater collaboration at many different levels'. In the health service we are seeing the same top-down driven initiate. A recent (September 2000) policy document on managed clinical networks indicates the drive towards networks stems from the American experience and especially the 'realisation that the range of needs of humans is infinite and continuous in comparison to the capability of traditional organisations to treat need which is infinite and discontinuous' (NHS 2000).

## Implications for the health service

Clearly the industrial network model is highly relevant, but caution is needed in applying it to health care. It needs to be made specific to the case, with appropriate modifications and changes. The basis for transfer and interaction (communication only, collaboration only, trading only or a mixture) needs to be explored and especially the limits: what we can use, what we cannot. For instance, the definition of managed clinical networks (Scottish Office 1999), comprising linked primary, secondary, tertiary care, is entirely in keeping with definition of industrial networks as value chain activities, comprising not only horizontally, but also vertically, integrated activities.

Although the managed clinical networks initiative is strong, and initial attempts at implementation in Scotland have met with some success, there are some key tensions between the network model presented here and that envisaged in various NHS policy documents, which bear examination if the initiative is to be successful. The basis of these tensions may be focused on the following paragraph from the Scottish Office (1999, p 47):

> . . . some concern was expressed during the Review that the term network can suggest 'non-organisation', loose 'wooly' constructs without authority, defined responsibilities or ability to exert control. Such constructs would be totally unacceptable; clinical networking cannot be a 'free for all', and issues of patient safety, confidentiality, risk management, individual accountability and professional responsibility must be defined and reconciled. It is to underline the importance of these considerations that the Review, in promoting networking, favours the use of the term managed clinical network and sees the concept of a lead clinician as having central importance.

Undoubtedly healthcare networks face a different set of pressures and constraints to a business network, and the report quoted above acknowledges this. At the same time, it is a mistake to dismiss the importance of network key features out of hand. Business networks are characterised by the features described above. The point that must be stressed is that these features are all **interrelated**. Adaptability is to a great extent the product of the unique set of relationships that hold between network actors. These relationships arise as a result of freely made decisions about whether or not to collaborate. They are not the product of a central source of authority imposing an imperative to collaborate on the actors involved. The decision to collaborate is made in the context of more than one potential interaction. It is also influenced by the presence of a social context, i.e. interactions between actors do not take place in a vacuum, they are social events witnessed by others. The culture and social milieu also influence the decisions made. On the basis of these decisions, resources and knowledge are shared and collaboration and interdependence are developed.

Networks and network 'behaviours' are a product of the key features. There is no suggestion here that networks are characterised by terms such as 'non-organisation' or 'woolly' constructs. That is to misunderstand what networks are. However, 'authority, defined responsibilities and the ability to exert control' are concepts that belong to a different form of organisation, a more centralised model. In moving towards a network form, different dynamics come into play and operate between network actors, their decisions to collaborate are based on a different set of reasons. That is not the same thing as 'non-organisation'. There are some who believe that the network form of organisation is really a more open and honest appraisal of human economic behaviour and an admission that business is made up of people who make decisions for personal, social and cultural reasons, as well as rational and economic ones. Furthermore, some believe that this has been the case all along, but centralised models of organisation based on mechanical models of physical systems have come to hold sway in the sphere of social organisation. These 'traditional' models based on ideas of prediction and control provide the illusion that people are being managed and behave rationally. Network models acknowledge that decisions to act are complex and are not effectively managed from top down every time. The question is what provision must be made in adopting the model for the health service that satisfies the requirements of that sector.

The adoption of a network model is able to confer a number of distinct and unique advantages in terms of health service provision:

- A flexible, tailored service
- An effective pooling and utilisation of resource
- Collaboration between diverse groups and communities of care
- Integration among primary, secondary and tertiary care
- Containment of health costs.

In transferring the model from a business to a health service context, four key tensions are identified as significant:

### Accountability vs network collective responsibility

A significant feature of networks is the idea of collective endeavour, the pulling together of individual value-added activities to meet a commonly accepted goal. This has the effect of creating a sense of collective accountability which nurtures and strengthens relationships between network actors. There is an important divergence between this aspect of networks and the idea of individual accountability and traceability. These are an especially significant element of NHS management and operation, especially important where issues of human life are concerned. Here these two are recognised as being to an extent in opposition.

## Management centrally vs self-organisation

One of the key features of the business network model above is that of self-organisation, meaning that power is not centralised in any one area in the network, and that no one actor or set of actors has the ability to exercise control over the behaviour of the others. Relationships taking the form of exchanges and collaboration are the product of a choice freely made by network actors. The idea of managed clinical networks is in some respects a challenge to this key feature. Successful business networks studied are characterised to an extent by the existence of central nodes. These nodes act as information and knowledge conduits, as agents. Their role is to gather information about the environment within which the network is embedded and the requirements of that environment, and to disseminate this information in the network. In some cases this takes the form of the agents mobilising the 'right' mix of network actors to develop and provide a response to the perceived environment need. This is a completely different role to the one suggested by the Scottish paper (Scottish Office 1999) in which a lead clinician is suggested as taking a central role. The question must be asked whether that role will impact decisions and relationship development in the network adversely or not. That will depend to a great extent on the culture and disposition of network actors – previous experiences, perceptions, assumptions, etc.

## Standards in practice vs improvisation

Network behaviour is characterised by its flexibility and adaptability. Improvisation is an important part in this, almost by definition. Flexibility is the ability to respond to unpredicted and hitherto unknown circumstances using whatever resources are available. To achieve this, network actors need not only to be able to improvise but also to have the capability to offer more than the required diversity of behaviours and responses. They need to have excess diversity within them, so that they can respond to unknown and unpredicted circumstances. At the same time, health service provision has to offer some levels of standards in practice. Although each patient is unique and requires unique care, there must also be some understanding of the necessary levels and standards of care. The question is recognising when to go beyond these standards.

## Long term vs short term

The time frame for any new initiative is very important. Networks are on the whole more suited to longer-term perspectives. The time it takes to establish a network should not be underestimated. Networks are not simply a different method, they involve a different mind-set and attitude, and these take a long time to establish fully. On the other hand, although in the shorter term network behaviour may appear to be suboptimal (and this includes the area of costs), this is because their benefits are realised in a longer-term perspective. In the shorter term, it is possible to have a certain degree of confidence that things will remain the same, and on this basis to create structures and organisations that will support the provision of services in an optimal manner. In the longer term, this certainty is lost, with the result that it is not possible to optimise systems on the same basis. In these unpredictable situations, flexibility is more appropriate with a resultant loss of optimality. It is not feasible to assume that process optimisation is always the most desirable outcome in a longer-term context.

In conclusion, the adoption of the network model in the health sector cannot be assumed to be a straightforward transfer from a business context to a health context. The following key points are drawn as a set of concluding remarks:

- There is a need to redefine what is meant by a network and network behaviours in the context of the health service and the environment within which it is embedded.
- There is a need to be clear about what networks are good for, why they have been enthusiastically drawn upon in the business context and, as the flip side to this, to accept what they are not good for. Networks are not necessarily a panacea, any more than any organisational form is, and if applied improperly they can lead to increased confusion, disillusionment and failure.
- The key network features of adaptability and flexibility have to be reinterpreted for an NHS context. In the business sphere they are relevant to the drives towards globalisation and mass customisation. What does this mean, however, in a health service context?
- There is a need to resolve the key tensions identified above, realising that each of them leads to compromise. They need to be redefined in line with NHS expectations, needs and reality.
- The role of the patient needs to be brought forward as a crucial partner in the process, an important network actor.
- Barriers and constraints need to be properly identified and understood. Some of these may be easy to surmount, others may not. One of the most important and insidious is the issue of power and the history of power holding in the existing organisation. It must be recognised that the individuals who have held these places will feel threatened and will not easily yield their power.
- Finally, the importance of the individual's decision-making process about whether to participate in the network, to collaborate, cannot be ignored. In simple terms the key question being asked is 'What's in it for me?'. Incentives and performance measures must reflect desirable network behaviours.

In brief, the model must be modified somewhat, but it must be accepted that, in modifying it, some of the characteristic features and behaviours of networks are compromised. At its best, this may lead to a new model relevant specifically to the health sector. At worst, it may lead to disillusionment with network models, unless the issues and tensions above are carefully considered, understood and accepted from the start.

## *References*

Alter C & Hage J (1993). *Organizations Working Together*. Sage Library of Social Research, no. 191, London: Sage

Axelrod R (1984). *The Evolution of Co-operation*. New York: Basic Books

Axelsson B & Easton G, eds (1992). *Industrial Networks – A New View of Reality*. London: Routledge

Becattini G (1990). The Marshallian industrial district as a socio-economic notion. In Pyke F, Becattini G, Sengenberger W (eds) *Industrial Districts And Inter-Firm Co-operation In Italy*. Geneva: International Institute of Labour Studies

Best M (1990). *The New Competition – Institutions of Industrial Restructuring*. Cambridge: Polity Press

Biggiero L (1999). Markets, hierarchies, networks, districts: a cybernetic approach. *Human Systems Management* **18**(2), 71–86

Blau P (1964). *Exchange and Power in Social Life*. London: John Wiley & Sons

Burt RS (1992). *Structural Holes: The social structure of competition*. Cambridge, MA: Harvard Business Press

Coro G & Grandinetti R (1999). Evolutionary patterns of Italian district networks. *Human Systems Management* **18**(2), 117–129

Department of Trade and Industry (1988). *Our Competitive Future – Building the Knowledge Driven Economy*. UK Government Competitiveness White Paper. London: DTI.

Farinelli F (1996). *Networks of Firms Confronting the Challenge of Globalisation: The Italian Experience*. IPTS Report, no. 7, September, pp 14–20

Gillies JM (2000). Industrial network adaptability: a complex systems based model, PhD thesis, Cranfield University

Grabher G (1993). Rediscovering the social in the economics of inter-firm relations. In Grabher G (ed.) *The Embedded Firm: On the socio-economics of industrial networks*. London: Routledge

Lazerson MH (1988). Organizational growth of small firms: an outcome of markets and hierarchies? *American Sociological Review* **53**, 330–342

Lazerson MH & Lorenzoni G (1998). *The Firms That Feed Industrial Districts: A Return To The Italian Source*. Working paper, Economics Faculty, University of Bologna

Lipnack J & Stamps J (1994). *The Age of the Network – Organising Principles for the 21st Century*. Essex Junction, VT: Oliver Wight Publications

Lipparini A & Sobrero M (1994). The glue and the pieces: entrepreneurship and innovation in small firm networks. *Journal of Business Venturing* **9**, 125–140

Marshall A (1890). *Principles of Economics*. London: Macmillan

NHS (2000). *Managed Clinical Networks*. London: NHS

Nohria N & Eccles RG, eds (1992). *Networks and Organisations – Structure, Form and Action*. Boston, MA: Harvard Business School Press

Powell WW (1990). Neither market nor hierarchy: network forms of organization. *Research in Organizational Behaviour* **12**, 295–336

Sabel CF (1986). Changing models of economic efficiency and their implications for industrialisation in the third world. In Foxley A, McPherson M, O'Donnell G (eds) *Development, Democracy and the Art of Trespassing*. Paris: University of Notre Dame Press

Scottish Office (1999). Department of Health, MEL(1999)10. *Introduction of Managed Clinical Networks Within the NHS in Scotland*. Management Executive Letter for the Scottish Health Executive, Edinburgh

Williamson OE (1975). *Markets and Hierarchies: Analysis and anti-trust implications*. New York: Free Press

# Chapter 7

# Networking care: the information management perspective

*Roderick Neame*

## Introduction

It is increasingly rare to find the entire range of care services, facilities and personnel required for the diagnosis and delivery of appropriate care in a manner consistent with best quality care protocols to every patient coexisting within a single enterprise. Even a relatively uncomplicated patient case will probably require the services of physicians, surgeons and allied health professionals across primary and secondary care. More complicated cases, such as cancer patients, are likely to require access to complex imaging and radiation technologies, specialised protocols and procedural skills, oncologists, palliative specialists and much more. Few organisations and enterprises, particularly those located away from major population centres, will be able to justify the investment in all these services and, where they do, they may find themselves too far away from many of their catchment population to be able readily to serve their needs. Therefore the probability of all the required services being available in a local institution becomes decreasingly likely.

The future of health care dictates that, as the emphasis on early detection and treatment increases, so there will increasingly frequently be a need to arrange access to services quickly, and in a co-ordinated way, at the same time as accommodating the wishes and care preferences of the patients, who may themselves reject some options on the basis of location, convenience, cost or other considerations.

In addition, there is a growing imperative that all those caring for the same patient are able to share the same patient record. Where a patient is moved between enterprises, there may be practical impediments to actually achieving meaningful transfers of patient records and information based in significant part on the incompatibilities of the record storage systems in use. In the absence of a shared record, there are serious difficulties in achieving integrity and continuity of care, leading not infrequently to adverse interactions between therapies: it would appear from many published studies that serious illness and even death may be a not uncommon consequence of such dis-integrity.

As a consequence there is a growing requirement for *networking* of care services. The *care network* comprises many service provider units and organisations, each of which are able to offer some services, and between them they are able to provide all the required services to care even for the most complex of cases. Where feasible it is likely that patients will prefer to receive care services at local institutions because these will be more convenient for them, even if for some specific services they may have to travel to another more distant location; the alternative of compelling patients to travel to the more distant location for all their care needs, even though some could be provided locally (and perhaps more quickly and more cost-effectively), is unlikely to be appealing to patients and is certainly not a patient-centred strategy.

This chapter outlines a conceptual approach to both of these issues based on an architecture that is both application and platform independent. The concepts are at present being tested in a small pilot initiative.

## Background

It is common to find that patients are essentially held 'captive' within a care enterprise or group of business entities. Typically in the UK, this arises where a patient is referred from a primary care clinic to 'the' local district general hospital, irrespective of the length of wait that this may entail, and often indeed irrespective of the performance and suitability of the services that it can offer to meet the care requirements of the patient. In North America a similar situation applies where an insurer may endeavour to keep the patient within a network of preferred providers and facilities. These arrangements are driven by commercial or other considerations, and have little to do with providing the best possible care to the patient in ways that best fit their preferences and requirements; indeed they may actually prove to be to the detriment of best quality patient care where services provided may not be premium quality.

It could be argued that such a restricted pattern of patient movements is for the best – that the integrity and continuity of care services to the individual can be better maintained within a single enterprise, even if this means that the services provided to the patient are in some instances suboptimal. Sadly there is all too often some actual basis for this, because the information management systems of secondary care enterprises and their neighbouring primary and community care services may be unable to support shared care arrangements. However, in the increasingly client-centred ('patient-focused') atmosphere that is now beginning to drive the healthcare delivery system, such an argument is self-evidently unacceptable. The solution to this issue is not to restrict patient access to facilities and services because of these shortcomings, but to enable the patient to choose the most appropriate, convenient, timely and cost-effective services, and to drive forward a strategy whereby these are all fully supported with the required information and, of course, attended by the appropriate security and personal information privacy infrastructure.

Various initiatives have been piloted whereby certain clinics in the community have been set up so as to be able to access and operate the appointments booking and admissions systems (PAS) of a specific hospital. Although this is a step forward in one sense, it is a step in a direction that does not facilitate the necessary following step(s) for care networking as described above.

However, this does not meet a large part of the real needs. For networked care to function it must be possible to book appointments at and/or admit patients to *any* appropriate facility, and to do this from *any* clinical setting, whether in the primary or secondary sector, in full knowledge of availability/waiting list conditions, etc. at all of them. The traditional approach to achieving meaningful data interchange between systems has been to create two bespoke interfaces (one in each direction) between each requesting system and each receiving system; the number of interfaces required for this architecture to function approximates the square of the number of systems involved [in fact $n(n-1)$], therefore incurring unacceptable expense as the numbers of systems becomes large – not to mention that, each time one system is altered or upgraded, all interfaces to and from it [totalling $2(n-1)$] need to be revised accordingly.

## Requirements for networking care

As reasoned above, any solution that effectively acts by providing no more than a remote access function for selected functions of one specific secondary care system is *not* what is required to support the networking of care. The required solution using the same generic access software and routine has to enable the referring practitioner, with his or her patient, whether booking from primary or secondary care, to arrange appropriate appointments at any convenient institution offering the needed care services within an acceptable timeframe.

Further, the networking of care requires that there should be a way of creating a shared patient record that is accessible, with the patient's consent, from any authorised provider location across the whole of primary or secondary care.

In practical terms the key goals are, therefore:

- to be able to identify the persons concerned – doctor and patient – in a way that means the same to all parties
- to be able to access and book appointments for the required service(s) offered by any service provider organisation from any referring service
- to be able to create a secure patient-centred record of the key data gathered and care provided that is accessible from any of the care services/locations involved by a duly authorised and authenticated person.

The key obstacles, on the other hand, are not only that there is variable penetration, use and functionality of the electronic systems for use in primary and secondary care, but also that these comprise a myriad of incompatible systems, specifically in terms of the ways they:

- identify patients, using their own internal unit record numbering and referencing systems

- manage appointments using their own proprietary patient administration systems (where electronic scheduling is used at all)
- store encounter data (clinical and administrative) using their own record data-sets, formats, coding and security.

The fact that many systems make use of different hardware, operating systems and communications protocols is no longer a barrier to meaningful data interchange, although the absence in many older systems of useful interfaces for data import/export can present a relative problem.

This diversity of systems is, in itself, healthy – at least potentially. It means that there is a wide range of alternative approaches to managing the information needs of the user. If users select carefully a system or systems that best meet their needs, structural and functional organisational arrangements, the variety of systems means that there is choice in the marketplace and that some solutions will probably better meet the requirements of each unit than others. Put another way, any attempt to impose a monolithic, centrally selected, single system is likely to be counterproductive, a view that is based in part on recent history of such initiatives (e.g. the 'single system for GPs' in the early to mid-1980s) as well as on the progressive 'privatisation' (often as a consequence of incipient collapse) worldwide of most of the state-owned health information management systems. The point is, therefore, that heterogeneity in internal enterprise information management and systems is inevitable and must therefore be accommodated in the solution proposed.

This predicates that the solution is based primarily on information engineering, defining data-sets and messages, and seeking the lowest common denominator for meaningful data interchange, rather than on technical engineering (e.g. standardising patient administration systems). This approach preserves the existing investment in legacy systems without impacting any arguments locally for or against upgrading them: it leaves users free to organise their internal information management in ways that best suit their business and clinical needs.

Rather than standardising the patient administration systems themselves, which, as outlined above, is not an appropriate way forward, what this approach does suggest is that there should be a move towards defining a standard interface to all local patient master indexes (LPMIs), local services schedulers (LSSs) and local event data records (LEDRs) systems. The issue is to determine the nature of these interfaces, which requires a further elucidation of the solution proposed.

## A proposed solution architecture

Inevitably in this era of networking technology, the only practical and generic solution to the problem lies in the use of web-enabled technology. In effect what is required is that all the proprietary LPMIs and LSSs from the participating enterprises should be able to interact with an open and standardised web-based regional patient master index (WRPMI) and web-based regional services scheduler (WRSS). In other words, when individuals access and use each of these systems, there is effectively a seamless interface through the internal applications into an external regional 'web-ised' equivalent. The regional systems will comprise a 'super-set' of all the local systems: they may contain fields that not every local system has, in which case these additional fields will be displayed only on systems that support that specific data-set.

The solution to the patient-centred record of care can also be addressed using web-enabled technology. Each care event gives rise to a record (e.g. encounter notes, pathology results, operation notes, etc.) which is stored internally in whatever proprietary form is used by the originating system. An interface is required to create the same record, or an edited subset of it, in mark-up language (HTML, XML, etc.). In various domains, and particularly that of cancer care, 'minimum' data-sets (MDSs) are being agreed for each event type in the care pathway: these will comprise the base for the shared care record. The 'original' record will, of course, be stored exactly as before within the local information system, but the web-enabled record for sharing can then be stored in a location to be agreed between the parties. Storage locations will include, for example, enterprise-owned web-servers, commercial servers, etc., but, perhaps most significantly, they can include personal internet-based 'security deposit boxes', which are controlled by and can only be opened and read by the patient or by others to whom the patient provides the access key and/or encryption algorithms. This addresses the concerns about protecting the privacy of personal information, placing it within the control of the patient as required by international and European law. Diagrammatically this can be illustrated as in Figure 7.1.

Where patients must be triaged according to urgency in order to determine whether routine or accelerated appointments should be offered, an agreed data-set is collected. This can be analysed according to rules or patterns determined by the service(s) concerned and the online booking made sooner or later depending on the outcome of that triage.

## Discussion

The inevitable reality of the evolution of care services in the context of funding limitations is that not every local hospital will have all the care services required for all types of patients, perhaps not even for a simple majority of patients. The effective collaboration between primary and community and secondary care services, which can be achieved only where there is adequate sharing of patient care information, is increasingly vital in order to provide a more patient-focused care service that can thereby assure continuity and integrity of care in a convenient and cost-effective way. The imperative to move towards networking of care services seems to be widely ignored at present, perhaps in some cases as a result of lack of recognition and in other cases of inability to see how to address the problem.

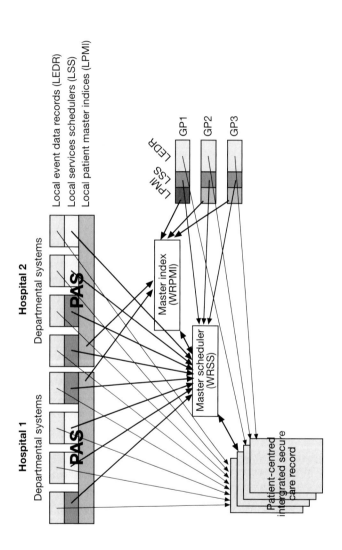

**Figure 7.1** Schematic arrangement and diagram of links between local and regional identifier, scheduler and records systems, over all of which a security layer is implemented. The integrity of the two links, shown as bold double-headed arrows, is crucial to this approach to integration of legacy care systems.

In many secondary care enterprises, the guiding philosophy behind information systems acquisition and development seems to be based on an 'island-thinking' model, which all but ignores the need for networked care or shared information. Institutions are seeking to extend the reach of their proprietary hospital information systems to primary care on a pilot basis without recognising or accepting that the architecture and technology that this implies inevitably ensures that the pilot is obsolescent before it starts. A less charitable interpretation might be that they are seeking to use proprietary technology to 'lock-in' their local primary care providers and endeavouring to tie them to using only their referral services.

Although clearly it is possible to develop a different interface and technology for every type of referral and for every different care institution, such a scheme would be impossible to implement in primary care. If the system is to be of value to doctors and patients alike, what is required is a single simple interface to all services and for all types of referrals.

Such a browser-based pilot has now been started in Kent by the Kent Cancer Services, and it is hoped that this will prove the functionality and utility of the approach and technology. The initial phase of the pilot is designed to test just the booking system; development of the patient-centred integrated care record must await an extension of the project. The pilot is limited to rapid access referrals for patients suspected of having certain cancers (breast, colorectal, lung, urological) from a small number of primary care settings to a limited number of hospital clinics. However, there is no limit to the numbers of GPs, hospital clinics and types of referrals that can be managed within this generic architecture.

When implemented, this pilot system will enable a primary care physician identifying a patient who seems to require an accelerated appointment to invoke a standard web browser to access the system server over the internet (or any other robust communications network). After selecting the type of referral (e.g. for suspected breast, colorectal cancer, etc.), the regionally agreed MDS is displayed as a form and the data-set collected. This completed form is sent to the server where it is analysed and stored; if the triage analysis suggests the probability of cancer, the scheduler for the regional rapid access clinics is invoked and displays a listing of clinic locations, clinic consultants and clinic dates; if the analysis indicated that this is not an urgent case, only a routine appointment will be offered. The doctor, with the patient, opts to fix one parameter (e.g. location) and a matrix of available consultant clinics and dates (i.e. care service sessions) is displayed; selection of any one of these unique care sessions displays the available appointment times, and selection of a time from this list makes the appointment. The system then prints a 'ticket' for the patient to take away: the ticket gives full information about the appointment, how to prepare for it, how to get there, what to do on arrival, what will happen and who to contact in case of concerns. There is also a personal 'key' on the ticket, which in future will permit patients to access (and to authorise others to access) their personal care records within this environment.

## Conclusion and the way forward

In this chapter the author argues that networking of care services and shared care will become the norm for most patients if it is not already. Existing information management systems are poorly aligned with this requirement, and many enterprises have yet to come to grips with what it means in information management terms.

The solution proposed involves the development of a generic web-enabled regional (or national) PMI for common identification of patients, and a regional encounter master scheduler for online booking of appointments. These will be interfaced with existing primary and secondary care systems such that the PMI appears to be an extension of their internal PMI, and that appointments can be made online, which are immediately passed through to the relevant service scheduler (often integrated into a PAS).

All care events within this framework will give rise to an encounter MDS, increasingly a data-set that has been agreed between the participants. These MDSs, often with additional data or notes, form the basis of a web-enabled patient-centred record of care. The elements of this record can be stored in any agreed location, and encrypted if so desired; the author's preference is for the use of personal web-based security deposit boxes that can be opened only by the patient with their personal key, or by those authorised by the patient using his or her key.

# Chapter 8

# Accountability of managed clinical networks

*Tera Younger*

## Introduction

This chapter looks at accountability issues for managed clinical networks in general and with particular reference to cancer services, drawing on experience with developing five managed clinical networks for cancer services in London. The chapter begins with a summary of the evolution of the managed clinical network model of organisation and service delivery, definitions of managed clinical networks and functions assigned to networks by various groups. This provides a context for examining the roles and responsibilities for which networks are to be held accountable and the behavioural changes required for networks to exercise the various dimensions of their accountability.

## Background

### Early work in developing the concept of managed clinical networks

The 1995 Calman–Hine Report (Department of Health 1995) was considered as a model for the later National Service Frameworks (NSF), and set the stage for 'networks' being the key organising principle for the diagnosis and treatment aspects of cancer services across England and Wales. In describing the recommended new structure for cancer services, the Report says:

> The new structure should be based on a network of expertise in cancer care reaching
> from primary care through Cancer Units in district hospitals to Cancer Centres . . .
> to ensure that the benefits of specialised care are available to all patients either close
> to their homes or, when necessary, by referral to special Centres. The integration of
> these three levels of care with each other . . . should provide a comprehensive cancer
> service . . . using local expertise and agreed protocols . . . . [T]his network is one of
> proficiency and not of buildings.

When it was published, the Calman–Hine Report was considered somewhat revolutionary for several reasons: first, because the internal market approach to the organisation and delivery of NHS services at that time focused on devolution of decision-making to local bodies, whereas the Calman–Hine Report was a *national planning framework*; second, because the internal market focused on competition between healthcare organisations as the principal lever for improving the quality and cost-effectiveness of services, whereas Calman–Hine's organisational model was one of *integration and partnership* between institutions and levels of care across organisational boundaries.

During the first phase of implementation of the Calman–Hine Report (1995–1999), the focus was primarily on the development and 'designation' (accreditation) of the acute care components of cancer using the 'hub-and-spoke' model of partnership networks – cancer centres (hubs) and cancer units (spokes) – for the common cancers. However, during the latter part of the 1990s, there was growing recognition that, for full achievement of the integration of services envisioned in the Calman–Hine Report, the initial acute 'hub-and-spoke' model needed to develop into a broader and more organised 'network' model which can plan, organise and deliver cost-effective high-quality cancer services to a shared population across the entire patient care pathway. By transcending unhelpful barriers between disciplines, professional groups and institutions, cancer networks can have the flexibility to draw on the collective resources of all of the component parts of the local cancer care system to meet changing needs and exercise accountability for the service effectiveness and responsiveness required in a modern NHS.

The 1997 White Paper, *The New NHS: Modern and Dependable*, called on the NHS to implement a model of health service organisation 'called "integrated care" based on partnership and driven by performance'. The Government established 'a new statutory duty for NHS trusts to work in partnership with other NHS organisations . . . in developing Health Improvement Programmes (HIMPs) under the leadership of the Health Authority . . . . The days of the NHS Trust acting alone without regard for others are over . . . . In an NHS based on partnership it will be increasingly important for the staff of NHS Trusts to work efficiently and effectively in teams within and across organisational boundaries'. However, the White Paper did not specifically use the term 'networks'.

It was the 1998 Scottish Executive *Acute Services Review Report* that provided much of the conceptual base for the growing interest in managed clinical networks as an alternative to the 'hub-and-spoke' model of care, featuring 'the sharing of patients, expertise and resources (across the entire patient pathway) rather than unidirectional centripetal flow'. The Report pointed out that 'the term "hub and spoke" can sometimes be unhelpful to the implied subordinate status of the "spoke" and the model does not readily reflect the key role of primary care in health services delivery'. The *Acute Services Review* concluded that the network model offers 'the best prospect for delivering high quality services which make optimal use of resources and offer more uniform access to patients'. The term 'managed clinical networks' was chosen deliberately to distinguish the recommended model from the notion of 'loose woolly constructs without authority, defined responsibilities or ability to exert control . . . . The managed clinical network can of course draw on elements of the "hub and spoke" as appropriate … [but] have other important connotations. For example, strategic investment in equipment would be driven by the needs of the network rather than the needs of any one hospital . . .'.

## Experience of development of managed clinical networks for cancer services in London

In London, by 1999 each of the five geographical sectors had begun to recognise the importance of developing their cancer networks to formalise joint management structures for the 'hub-and-spoke' cancer networks that had evolved around the five London cancer centres. This development work included convening network tumour-specific groups and starting work to varying degrees on network-wide structures and strategic plans. These represented the first steps in adopting the networking approach to the delivery of cancer services in our region.

The *Modernisation Plan for the NHS in London, 1999–2002* (Department of Health 1999), identified cancer as one of the priority areas for development of a London-wide service strategy. One of the key elements of this service strategy was to 'agree London-wide core principles for the roles and responsibilities of the five London cancer networks . . . to enable the networks to take on an increasing role in driving the continuing development of Calman-Hine'. To take this forward, a regional conference was held on 30 November 1999 'to explore key features of cancer networks and their role in improving the delivery and outcomes of services for [the London] population' as proposed in a draft discussion paper. In inviting people to this conference, the Regional Director, Nigel Crisp, indicated that:

> We regard managed clinical networks as a key feature of implementing our plan for modernising and improving NHS services in London. Since our five Cancer Networks are at a more mature state of development than perhaps in other service areas, we would like to see further development of Cancer Networks . . . as a forerunner to other work on clinical networks in other specialties.

Following feedback from the conference, the draft discussion paper setting out the specifications for further development of managed clinical networks for cancer services was finalised in February 2000 and transmitted to local NHS organisations by the Regional Director, along with a request that each of the five London cancer networks develop draft 2-year strategies by April 2000. These draft strategies were reviewed by the Regional Office against the agreed specifications; comments were sent back to each network; revised strategies were received in autumn 2000; and all but one revised strategy was 'signed off' by the Regional Office on 1 February 2001. In line with the London Region's new strategic framework for improving palliative care services, supportive and palliative care networks are beginning to be established across London, which will link with the cancer networks and with networks for other diseases (e.g. coronary heart disease, HIV/AIDs).

## The NHS Cancer Plan and National Manual of Cancer Services Standards

The publication of *The NHS Cancer Plan* in September 2000 (Department of Health 2000d) established a national requirement for the development of cancer networks in all English regions as 'the organisational model for cancer services to implement this Cancer Plan'. Key functions and milestones are set out in the plan. Thus, if there was a question in some areas about *whether* networks would be the organisational model for cancer services for the future, that question has now been answered. Thirty-four cancer networks have been established across England. The national *Manual of Cancer Services Standards* (NHS Executive 2000b), published in December 2000, includes standards for cancer network management arrangements and key deliverables to implement *The NHS Cancer Plan*. Further details of these standards are discussed later.

## Purpose and goals of managed clinical networks

The principal objectives hoped to be achieved by managed clinical networks are summarised below. Managed clinical networks offer:

> . . . the best basis for equitable, rational and sustainable acute services, are flexible and capable of evolution, and allow greater emphasis to be placed on service performance and effectiveness . . . . [The network model's goals are]: promoting equity for patients; providing a stimulating environment for staff in which there is equal access to resources; facilitating multidisciplinary working, skill enhancement and professional development; strengthening training programmes for all staff; and fostering research and development.
>
> The Scottish Office (1998)

The managed clinical network model is intended to overcome the difficulty with the 'hub-and-spoke' model in which:

> . . . clinical care in the spoke is managed by one management team and care in the hub is managed by another. There is no pressure on these organisations to integrate the way services are provided in order to offer a better service to the patient. [Managed Clinical Networks are intended] to encourage a change in the way services are managed . . . to integrate the way services are provided in order to offer a better service to the patient.
>
> Burns (1998)

> Adoption of a networked approach for the delivery of acute services – groups of services and sites, working within a single system, with common management . . . may be the only approach [to allow the health care system to respond effectively to changes introduced by the Government's White Papers] which will combine the scale required for economic and quality performance, with the continuing local delivery of many services.
>
> Newchurch & Co. (1999)

The purpose of managed care [delivered through managed clinical networks] is to encourage greater accountability from the providers of health care, principally doctors, for the resources they consume on behalf of patients.

Hunter (1999)

The objective is to improve quality and ensure the same high level of care is available to all cancer patients by bringing all the service providers together into a unified system.

Department of Health (2000a)

Through cancer networks, services can be planned across the care pathway for cancer patients with resources targeted where they are most needed to serve the cancer need of their local population – which may not be in the local hospital. Seamless care is promoted and alliances can develop to help reduce the risk of cancer, through action on smoking and diet.

Department of Health (2000d)

To ensure that all commissioners and providers of cancer care, the voluntary sector and local authorities within the network work effectively together to deliver high quality care . . . . To ensure that cancer services are managed and organised effectively to support high quality care.

Department of Health (2000e)

. . . at this early stage, the benefits are perceived to be: a mechanism for developing partnerships, opportunities to remove obstacles and blocks at service interfaces because of organisational boundaries, . . . improving services and equality of provision and access, . . . opportunities for better value for money.

Department of Health (2000c)

Although the emphasis may be slightly different in each of these statements about the purpose of networks, the themes are similar: to promote greater equity in the availability of high-quality, seamless and clinically/cost-effective care to a shared patient population by bringing all elements of the provision of services into a single system across the entire patient pathway.

## Definitions of managed clinical networks

The following are the definitions of NHS managed clinical networks that appear in the various reports discussed above:

. . . linked groups of health professionals and organisations from primary, secondary and tertiary care, working in a coordinated manner, unconstrained by existing professional and Health Board boundaries, to ensure equitable provision of high quality clinically effective services throughout Scotland.

The Scottish Office (1999)

. . . a 'virtual service organisation' comprising a linked group of professionals and organisations working across primary, community, secondary and tertiary care to ensure equitable and cost effective provision of the highest possible standard of cancer care to a population defined by their pattern of service used rather than place of residence . . . link(ed) into those involved with prevention and health promotion, patient information and advocacy.

Department of Health (2000a)

Cancer Networks . . . will bring together health service commissioners (health authorities, primary care groups and trusts) and providers (primary and community care and hospitals), the voluntary sector, and local authorities to deliver a comprehensive cancer service across the patient pathway. Each network will typically serve a population of around one to two million people.

Department of Health (2000d, 2000e)

As with the goals attributed to managed clinical networks, although the precise wording of these three definitions varies somewhat, their sense is essentially the same.

## Functions of managed clinical networks

The principal functions that managed clinical networks are being expected to perform are listed below. The 'letter' after each function shows which of the reports discussed above includes this function in its list of network responsibilities: The Scottish Office (1999) (S); Department of Health (2000a) (L); and Department of Health (2000d, 2000e) (NCP). In England, the NCP requirements now supersede previous regional requirements:

- Manage continuing implementation of the Calman–Hine Report (L).
- Implement *The NHS Cancer Plan* (including achievement of the Plan's targets and related guidance such as the Improving Outcomes series and NICE guidance on drugs) (NCP).
- Develop a cancer network 2-year strategic plan for the development of network services in accordance with national, regional and HIMP priorities (draft spring 2000; final autumn 2000) following a baseline assessment of current service configuration (L).
- Develop a 3-year 'service delivery plan' to develop all aspects of cancer services – prevention, screening, diagnosis, treatment, supportive care and specialist palliative care services (autumn 2001) following a baseline assessment of workforce, education and training, facilities and palliative care (summer 2001) (NCP).

- Develop a proposal to obtain formal approval by local trusts and health boards for recognition of a new/existing network that incorporates a defined set of core principles (S).
- The strategic plans (L), 'service delivery plans' (NCP) and proposals for formal recognition (S) should be underpinned by:
  - workforce, education and training, cancer facilities, palliative care and NICE drug strategies (NCP)
  - defined service configuration that sets out which services will be delivered where and the connections between the different elements of the network (L, S) to achieve continuous quality improvement and cost-effective use of resources (both NHS and voluntary sector), including the future distribution of services, staffing and equipment, and introduction of high cost drugs across the network (L)
  - agreement by the constituent members of the network about their contributions to implementing the network strategy through the HIMP and SAFF process (NCP)
  - evidence of exploration of the network's potential for generating better value for money (S)
  - a clear statement of specific clinical and service improvements which patients could expect as a result of establishment of the network (S)
  - implementation of the Cancer Services Collaborative, Phase 2 (NCP).
- Define evidence-based patient pathways (L); guidelines for referral of patients to a given level of care (NCP).
- Ensure effective operation of network tumour-specific groups to agree network-wide clinical guidelines/protocols (L, NCP).
- Establish a quality assurance/audit programme to ensure compliance with national, regional and network standards of care (L, S) and to feed into the clinical governance programmes of constituent trusts and primary care groups/trusts (PCGs/PCTs) (L).
- Agree and conduct at least two network-wide audits per tumour site (NCP).
- Agree a list of clinical trials per tumour site into which patients may be entered (NCP); promote research opportunities (L, S), and establish agreed protocols for entering patients into clinical trials (L).
- Set standards for education and continuing professional training across the network (NCP, L, S); have an appropriate programme of continuous professional development in place for every member of the network (S).
- Have a clear policy on the effective dissemination of appropriate information to patients, developed in consultation with patient groups (L, S).
- Establish a plan for the collection and analysis of information across network sites that feeds into the quality assurance programme (L); a minimum data-set (using the national MDS when available) (NCP),

- Produce an annual report that can be used by constituent organisations to feed into their local clinical governance programmes (L) and also be made available to patients (S).
- Establish clear management arrangement to ensure accountability in delivering the above functions (NCP, L, S). The management structure should include the following elements:
  - specification of the accountabilities and involvement of service providers (chief executives and clinicians), commissioners (health authorities and PCGs/PCTs), voluntary sector and patient representation (NCP)
  - a network board/steering group/management group with a named chair (NCP, L); with managerial and clinical representation from health authorities, cancer centres and units, primary care community trusts, patients and the voluntary sector (L); with agreed terms of reference that include recognition, by chief executives of NHS trusts/health authorities in the network, of the management group as the body responsible for producing the network's 3-year 'service delivery plan' and underpinning strategies as required by *The NHS Plan* (NCP)
  - a network management team: lead clinician/clinical director (NCP, L), lead manager (NCP, L) and lead nurse (NCP)
  - network tumour site-specific groups agreed by network members to be the source of the network's clinical opinion on matters relating to their particular tumour site (NCP, L)
  - generic groups covering such areas as chemotherapy, information, primary care, patient representation and palliative care (NCP, L)
  - a single multidisciplinary network palliative care group which is responsible for developing a network-wide palliative care strategy and drug formulary (NCP).
- The network should provide the template and forum for agreeing a commissioning strategy for the network (NCP, L).
- The network board/steering group/management group should be recognised by the NHS trust and health authority chief executives in the network 'as the appropriate and final common pathway to channel business between commissioners and providers on issues relating to cancer services provided for the whole network and to coordinate providers' views to any interested parties outside the NHS on such services' (NCP).
- The network strategic plan should have the support of all commissioners that purchase services for network residents so that there is consistent commissioning by health authorities, PCGs and PCTs (L).

## Essential characteristics of managed clinical networks: a summary

What does the above analysis of the historical evolution, goals, definitions and functions of managed clinical networks imply about their essential characteristics? These could be summed up as follows:

1  Partnerships
2  Emphasising connections rather than isolation and self-sufficiency
3  Virtual service organisations
4  Shared sovereignty with member organisations
5  Requiring the skills of a diplomat rather than that of an entrepreneur in a market-based system (Ferlie & Pettigrew 1996)
6  Actively managed not just consensual or collegial
7  Not just cancer centre driven but representing the perspectives of all members (DeWitt 2000).

## Implications for accountability of managed clinical networks

Having established the context within which NHS managed clinical networks will be expected to function, and the key organisational characteristics of networks that define the strengths and complexities of the structures within which they will have to function, we can now turn to an examination of how networks can exercise accountability – and be held accountable – for implementing their responsibilities effectively. If the passage by Hunter quoted above rings true – that the very purpose of the managed network model is to improve accountability of the wider healthcare system – then the accountability of networks themselves is a key issue.

This section will examine *what* managed clinical networks are accountable for and *to whom* they are accountable; offer suggestions about *how* they can exercise that accountability; identify things that will *test* a network's accountability; provide *examples* of methodologies that networks have used to exercise accountability; and consider what *assistance* might be useful to networks in developing their accountability skills and programmes. This section focuses primarily on issues involving the accountability of managed clinical networks for cancer services.

### What are networks accountable for?

The answer to this question is relatively clear. Networks are accountable for delivering effectively on the programme of functions listed above under 'Functions of managed clinical networks'. As summed up by the National Cancer Director (Department of Health 2001a) this means 'planning, implementing and monitoring'.

## To whom are networks accountable?

Networks are accountable to a number of constituencies:

1 The population they serve.
2 Their member organisations:
   – to develop consensus on network goals, strategies and work programmes across organisational boundaries, and on investment decisions needed by their member organisations to implement this consensus
   – to ensure fairness and transparency in making network decisions
   – to provide an environment in which clinical and managerial staff of member organisations can obtain professional satisfaction and continuing development.
3 Any other group to which the network decides to report (e.g. sector chief executive groups).
4 Neighbouring networks to ensure effective and fair decisions on cross-boundary issues.
5 The NHS Executive (through the Regional Office) for effective implementation of a major national government (NSF-like) policy.

This chapter was written before the current reorganisation of the NHS was announced (e.g. establishment of 28 strategic health authorities (SHAs), to replace the existing 100 health authorities, from April 2002, and abolition of NHS Executive Regional Offices from April 2003). Therefore, this section of the chapter does not address the changes that may occur under the new NHS structure. It has been suggested that cancer networks could be accountable to their SHA, to a lead PCT or to some remnant of the NHS Executive Regional Office. Presumably this question will be answered when the final version of *Shifting the Balance of Power in the NHS* is issued by the Department of Health in January to February 2002. (See Department of Health [2001c] for the consultation version of this document, issued in July 2001.)

## What do networks need to do to exercise their accountability effectively?

1 Networks need to establish effective management structures as outlined above.

   – The board/steering group/management group needs to have wide representation from network members so that it is perceived as a credible and legitimate planning and decision-making group, not dominated by any one organisation (e.g. the Cancer Centre) (R DeWitt, unpublished paper).
   – The experience in London, as well as the recommendation in *The NHS Cancer Plan*, is that close involvement of chief executives of health authorities and trusts, as well as provider lead cancer clinicians, is essential for the governing body to have managerial and clinical decision-making authority. Several models have emerged in London.

- Two network boards are chaired by health authority chief executives and also include all other health authority/trust chief executives and lead cancer clinicians.
- Another network board includes only one health authority chief executive as chair (as the other chief executives in the geographical sector has been designated to chair other networks) and representation from other network members.
- Two networks are chaired by health authority directors of public health, with health authority/trust chief executives included as members of the board.

  If all chief executives are not themselves members of the board, either they need to ensure that they delegate responsibility to the board for network decision-making or the board needs to have rapid access to whatever other group (e.g. chief executives group) is considered as the ultimate decision-making body for that geographical sector. The model of the first two network boards described above appears to have the greatest capacity at this time for effective and timely leadership and decision-making, but this model might not be sustainable in the long term as more disease-specific networks emerge. The next most desirable model would appear to be the middle one, chaired by one chief executive, with direct access to the entire chief executive group for that geographical sector (which might be viewed as an 'umbrella' network governing body).

- Networks need to establish as quickly as possible the management team outline above (lead clinician/clinical director, lead manager, lead nurse), recruiting people who have track records of good leadership skills. The NHS Executive has made national recurrent funding of £40k available to each of the 34 cancer networks to help in recruitment of this team (Department of Health 2000b). In London, Macmillan Cancer Relief has generously supplemented this NHS funding for the cancer network management teams. Experience with London cancer networks has been that dedicated lead managers/clinical directors have made a real difference in enhancing the network's ability to implement and monitor their agreed strategy and work programme.
- Studies of networks have noted that building an effective network is very time-consuming and requires a long, sustained process to develop trust and consensus among network members. Therefore, members of the network board and tumour-specific groups need to be given sufficient time by their employing organisations to devote to network responsibilities (Ferlie & Pettigrew 1996). Scotland has recommended that consultant job descriptions be modified for explicit recognition of participation on tumour-specific groups as part of the job; a similar approach could be taken with board members.

– Studies of network management bring out the contribution that network
champions and innovators can make to the development of effective network
governance and management structures. But there is also a downside to relying
too much on personal leadership because the network can be destabilised if
known players leave. Therefore, institutionalisation of the network governance
structure is important (Ferlie & Pettigrew 1996).

– Network boards need to establish effective governance systems that allow
them to monitor the implementation of their strategies and work programmes,
identify obstacles and address them (including problematic behaviour of
specific network members). A question has been raised about the extent to
which the network chair/board can be expected to control the behaviour of
network members; yet it is the chair/board who is likely to be held accountable
by other network members, the NHS Executive and patients for failure of the
network to deliver (Ferlie & Pettigrew 1996). Therefore, some mechanism for
dealing with such problems needs to be found. We have an example in London
where one network chair used the authority of the network to veto the unilateral
decision of one trust to add two new consultants without getting network-wide
support. Peer pressure from other network member organisations might be
another way of addressing this. Yet another mechanism might be feedback to
the clinical governance programme/board of the problematic organisation.

– Similarly, the network governance structure must be capable of helping to
strengthen a failing trust (or otherwise reconfigure services to work around
the quality problem) so that one trust's weaknesses do not de-stabilise the
entire network. We have seen several examples of this in London, where the
network's intervention to establish joint appointments and reconfigure services
has begun to make a difference in strengthening trusts that have difficulty in
meeting standards.

2 Networks need to obtain an explicit commitment from member organisations to
delegate some authority and resources to enable the network to deliver effectively
on its responsibilities. Several London network strategies identify this commitment
explicitly. Local clinical governance programmes should be asked to consider
making their organisation's effective participation in the network one of their
'success criteria'.

3 Building ownership for the network's strategies and work programme within
member organisations – both at board and middle management level – is also
essential (Ferlie & Pettigrew 1996). This is particularly important where the
network model has been 'imposed' in a 'top-down' fashion, as in cancer services
(both in London and now nationally). This may be why the South East Region
recommended, before issuance of *The NHS Cancer Plan*, that managed clinical
networks should not be mandatory but an option; however, the network model is
now required for cancer, and ways of developing ownership must be found.

The role that trust non-executive directors might play in building ownership for the network at local level should be explored.

4   Accountability for the quality of services can be implemented through network board/clinical director monitoring of tumour-specific group performance and through audit of compliance with tumour-specific group guidelines, with feedback to trust clinical governance programmes. Consideration should be given to modifying consultant job descriptions to require compliance with tumour group guidelines (*Manual of Cancer Services Standards*, Standard 10.1/21 – Department of Health 2000e).

5   The publication of an annual report for the network is another tool that can be used to document a network's accountability – to network members, including local clinical governance programmes. The annual report can be used to document the network's achievement and identity as a clinical whole, with the emphasis on patients and the patient pathway rather than institutions. The annual report can also be made available to patients as one way of assuring them 'of the objective and rigour of decisions made on their behalf' (Smith 1999).

## What situations can 'test' the effectiveness of a network's accountability mechanisms?

From the very outset of the London Region's initiative to develop its five cancer networks in 1999, 'network accountability' has been an issue. At the beginning, it was mostly a theoretical issue. To whom is the network accountable? How should the 'split' accountabilities of individual clinicians/managers to their statutory employing organisations and to the non-statutory 'virtual organisation' of the network be resolved? However, as the London cancer networks have become more operational, the accountability issues they raise have become more practical.

1   Situations that have proved the most 'testing' of networks' accountability thus far have involved service reconfiguration decisions – when tensions and power struggles between network members have come to the fore. Examples are: implementation of the national 'improving Outcomes Guidance for Gynaecological Cancers', which requires shifting most gynaecological cancer surgery from cancer units to the cancer centre; and rationalisation of services between multiple sites of a 'joint' cancer centre or a multi-site trust. Mechanisms adopted by networks to demonstrate 'fair' and 'transparent' network decision-making with respect to service reconfiguration have included public consultation and formal option appraisals, using external specialist evaluators against agreed formal criteria. Another technique being used by one network is to consider the reconfiguration of services for several tumour sites together, so that a trust that 'loses' services for one tumour type might 'gain' services for another. Both of these mechanisms are quire time-consuming, however. It remains to be seen whether, over time,

networks could make these configuration decisions in a more straightforward fashion using their own internal tumour groups or board structures to make these decisions. Thus far, tumour groups have found it difficult to make these decisions within the framework of their remit. The involvement of chief executives in making these difficult decisions has proved essential.

2  As noted above, other situations that 'test' network accountability mechanisms include a 'failing' trust; a trust/health authority that is reluctant to commit sufficient resources to implement network goals (e.g. implementation of agreed action plans to meet regional/national standards of quality care); and a trust that makes unilateral significant investment decisions (e.g. staffing, equipment, service configuration) without first obtaining network support. The earlier discussion of these 'tests' provides examples of some of the techniques that have been effective in addressing such issues.

3  Another situation that could 'test' network accountability is where a network member decides that it needs to give greater priority to other NHS Plan targets (e.g. waiting lists) than to the network's cancer strategy.

4  Finally, network accountability will be 'tested' by NHS Executive performance monitoring of a network's delivery on its cancer strategy and NHS Cancer Plan deliverables. Just as developing allegiance to networks requires different skills and behaviours on the part of network members, monitoring of network performance will require a different orientation from monitoring of individual institutions. Developing a good understanding of the network model will be important for those responsible for the performance monitoring process.

## What assistance might be useful to networks in developing their accountability skills and programmes?

1  Ferlie and Pettigrew (1996) note the role that network development programmes can play in helping network managers and clinicians develop the necessary skills and behaviours required for network versus single-institution management: trust, reciprocity, understanding, credibility, and ability to persuade, construct long-term relationships and deal with uncertainty and ambiguity. Network development programmes could also focus on helping network leaders develop approaches for dealing with the 'testing' situations discussed above. The national Cancer Action Team has run a series of network development events. Regional Offices have also sponsored network development programmes. Action learning sets might also provide a good forum for network development, to enable networks to learn from each other.

2  London networks have asked for assistance in understanding how to engage 'expert patient representatives' to help institutionalise a network culture in which the patient pathway and quality of patient care are at the centre – important in itself and also as a tool in getting network members to focus on a shared goal of improving care for 'patients' rather than on tensions between themselves.

3 The NHS Executive can play a role in reinforcing the importance of network-wide decision-making. In London, several 'levers' have been used in this way with respect to cancer networks:

– requiring that all business cases submitted (e.g. to the Regional Office) for approval of investment in new equipment/staff have the explicit support of the network board
– requiring an agreed network-wide proposal for the use of any new national funding (e.g. the £10m tranches of funding re specific cancers), pooling the allocations to the various health authority members
– empowering the network role in the new peer review process (to evaluate providers against the standards in the national *Manual of Cancer Services Standards*) by having the visiting team reports go to the networks for review and transmission to the Regional Office with a recommendation about the type of 'designation' (accreditation) decision that should be approved.

## For what things do clinicians/managers working in a network remain accountable to their employing organisations?

A discussion of network accountability would not be complete without attention to this question as well. The following points provide a suggested framework:

1 Staff working in each network would continue to be accountable to the organisation holding their contract of employment for performance-related issues. However, as suggested above, staff job descriptions could be revised to include relevant network accountabilities (e.g. the role of various staff on the network board, network tumour-specific groups, the obligation of clinicians to follow network clinical and patient pathway protocols) so that the employing organisation, in reviewing staff performance against these network responsibilities in their job descriptions, could actually reinforce staff accountability to the network.
2 The clinical governance programme of a trust member of the network would continue to be responsible for reviewing its organisation's performance in the round, including its contribution to the network. The network annual report could provide useful information here. Network boards could also communicate directly with trust clinical governance programmes about specific issues involving trust staff vis-à-vis the network.
3 If a clinician is involved in a potential 'serious untoward incident,' the trust medical director (not the network) would be responsible for addressing the issue.

## Conclusion

The 'blurring of organisational boundaries' (Smith 1999) inherent in the managed clinical network model results in a complex web of accountability for where there is no simple 'line management' recipe – as there would be in a hierarchical organisation.

However, this complexity does not make achieving accountability insurmountable, but rather makes it a challenging opportunity to improve the total system of care for patients. It is hoped that this chapter has provided a framework for considering network governance and accountability issues. Although this chapter has focused primarily on the experience with cancer networks, the principles should be applicable to managed clinical networks for other disease or service groups, although the 'environments' within which these other networks need to function will differ and present their own challenges (Flynn *et al.* 1996; Baker & Lorimer 2000; D O'Donoghue & J Scott 2000, unpublished paper).

## *References*

Baker CD & Lorimer AR (2000). Cardiology: the development of a managed clinical network. *British Medical Journal* **321**, 1152–1153

Burns H (1998). So . . . who wants to work in a spoke? *Journal of Integrated Care* **2** (editorial)

Department of Health (1995). *A Policy Framework for Commissioning Cancer Services: A Report by the Expert Advisory Group to the Chief Medical Officers of England and Wales* (Calman–Hine Report). London: Department of Health

Department of Health (1997) *The New NHS: Modern and Dependable*. London: Department of Health.

Department of Health, NHS Executive (1999). *The Modernisation Plan for the NHS in London, 1999–2002*. London: Department of Health

Department of Health, NHS Executive (2000a). *Managed Clinical Networks for Cancer Services*. London: Department of Health

Department of Health, National Cancer Director (2000b). Letter to Chairs of Cancer Network Management Groups and Regional Cancer Coordinators, Cancer Network Development Funding Allocation Process, 17 July, London

Department of Health, NHS Executive – South East (2000c). *Managed Clinical Networks*. London: Department of Health

Department of Health (2000d). *The NHS Cancer Plan*. London: Department of Health

Department of Health (2000e). *Manual of Cancer Services Standards*. London: Department of Health

Department of Health, National Cancer Director (2001a). The NHS Cancer Plan and the Role of Networks. Presentation at national conference on Networks, 10 January, London

Department of Health, NHS Executive (2001b). *Strategic Framework for Improving Palliative Care*. London: Department of Health

Department of Health (2001c). Shifting the Balance of Power within the NHS: Consultation document. London: Department of Health

Ferlie E & Pettigrew A (1996). Managing through networks: some issues and implications for the NHS. *British Journal of Management* **7**, 581–589

Flynn R, Williams G, Pickard S (1996). *Markets and Networks: Contracting in community health services*. Milton Keynes: Open University Press

Hunter DJ (1999). Integrated care. *Journal of Integrated Care* **3**, 155–160

Newchurch & Co. (1999). Acute transformation. In: *Healthcare After the White Paper*. London: Newchurch & Co.

The Scottish Office (1998). *Acute Services Review Report*. Edinburgh: NHS Management Executive

The Scottish Office (1999). Management Executive Letter, Introduction of Managed Clinical Networks Within the NHS in Scotland. Edinburgh: NHS Management Executive

Smith J (1999). Managed care: A framework for resource allocation in the NHS. *Journal of Integrated Care* **3**, 136–146

Chapter 9

# Clinical governance and accountability in cancer networks: data logging and data attribution

*Roger Cooley and Roger James*

## Background

### The NHS background

*Modernising NHS regulation using data collection*

Clinical governance in the NHS dates from a 1989 paper *Working for Patients* (Department of Health 1989) requiring doctors to adopt medical audit of their practice. Although audit has permeated the NHS over the last 12 years and included a variety of professional groups, adverse events surrounding clinical procedures continue to give rise to public concern, litigation and disciplinary procedures. There has been a recent perception that professional self-regulation (via the General Medical Council, Royal Colleges and traditional clinical governance) is inadequate.

In 2000, the Clinical Standards Board for Scotland published its *Quality Assurance and Accreditation Manual* which recommended a series of evidence-based clinical standards assessed by a process of external peer review. Standards have been produced for a series of secondary sector topics through the Scottish Intercollegiate Guideline Network (SIGN).

In 1999, the National Institute for Clinical Excellence (NICE) was established in England as a Special Health Authority to work closely with the Commission for Health Improvement (CHI) (NHS Executive 1999). NICE is responsible for analysing the evidence base for 'best practice' and recommends appropriate clinical policies and procedures. Audit performed by the CHI will direct clinical governance issues, regulation and revalidation (Buckley 1999).

In 2001, the National Patient Safety Agency was established as an independent body to collect and analyse data on adverse events in the NHS. Section 18 of the Health Act 1999 requires NHS institutions to put in place the framework for the improvement of health care and to provide the *evidence* or *data* that it is taking place.

### Attributability and electronic data transfer

Attributability for adverse events is a requirement of accountability and, ultimately, of effective management. In medicolegal investigations, accountability for the accuracy of the medical record is a central issue. Attributable data are signed and dated.

This implies that they were collected in real time, by an employee in a nominated post. Unattributable data are not verifiable at source, either as events in time or as events performed by an individual employee.

However, the entitlement to initiate life-threatening procedures in the NHS is increasingly based on complex data-sets logged electronically by a series of non-identified personnel. When all interested parties can access records from anywhere at any time, 'attributability' for an adverse event may be difficult to establish.

### National data-sets and epidemiology

In addition to regulation, *accurate and timely* audit of novel NHS procedures is also required for epidemiological reasons. The true cost-effectiveness of an intervention can be assessed only once it is in widespread use. There is a requirement to assess the *outcome* of any intervention in the specific UK health economy, using validated measures of cost and effectiveness. Assessment should be a dynamic process evaluating procedures in practice, in combination with other procedures.

## The cancer network background

### The development of cancer 'teams'

The 1995 Calman–Hine Report (Department of Health 1995) and subsequent commissioning guidance quote evidence that treatment for less common cancers should be based on a population rather than a hospital. Multidisciplinary teams (MDTs) with site specialisation are safer and more effective than individual, sporadic, clinical experiences. A cancer MDT consists of oncologists, surgeons, pathologists, radiologists and specialist nurses deciding treatment for individual patients. The MTD meeting fulfils many of the requirements of clinical governance, but has no statutory responsibility to collect data in an auditable form.

Each English cancer network is required to set up a series of tumour-specific groups (or disease-oriented groups, DOGs). Among other functions, the DOGs give advice to the network on clinical priorities for governance, investment and workforce planning. Governance priorities are dictated by the natural history of each cancer. It follows that the DOGs are at least partly accountable for clinically governing the data collection in each MDT meeting.

In NHS cancer networks the MDT meeting has emerged as the core of the most important aspect of data-based accountability because members of the MDT meeting jointly agree the most appropriate intervention for individual patients. MDT meetings have the explicit purpose of bringing the members' collective knowledge to bear on the medical aspects of a particular patient. They serve the primary purpose of decision-making, and in their archetypal form are attended by specified representatives in person, e.g. at a preoperative meeting to discuss intervention for a patient with colorectal cancer would include a surgeon, gastroenterologist, radiologist, pathologist, clinical oncologist, medical oncologist, specialist nurse and specialist palliative care representative. At such an MDT meeting, decisions would be taken about which of a range of possible treatment plans would be adopted. This would involve constituent decisions about: the 'intent' of the treatment, the modality of the treatment, secondary and tertiary treatment, and the name of the specialists responsible for the next phase of the treatment plan.

The MDT meeting forms a basis for clinical governance for several reasons. Networked cancer services in the NHS often mean that physical presence at meetings is increasingly difficult to organise, and this problem is exacerbated by staff shortages. The increased concern with the adequacy of professional self-regulation has given rise to a need for monitoring such meetings and attributable data.

## Data collection in cancer networks

Attributability for the accuracy of data collection has become an acute issue in NHS Cancer Services. The Gillis Report (2000) draws attention to deficiencies in the quality and timeliness of nationally collected cancer data and points out the need for greater co-ordination and collaboration among organisations. Trust chief executives are to be made ultimately accountable for the collection of *accurate and timely* cancer data, using nationally agreed data sets.

The Cancer National Service Framework has been standardised (*The Manual of Cancer Service Standards*: 'The Manual' – NHS Executive 2001). In April 2001 English cancer services were reconfigured into 34 networks and the self-assessment standards were published, assuming the implementation of this reconfiguration. 'The Manual' is designed to compare policies and procedures from network to network and record the names of employees responsible for aspects of care delivery. Auditors are expected personally to witness written policies. In summer 2001, all 34 English cancer networks were audited using the published standards and a peer-review process. It is likely that, in future, CHI will be responsible for the regular (2-yearly) audit. However, audit of implementation, process and outcome remains a feature of unconnected systems such as Cancer Registry Data Collection, high-level performance targets and clinical trials.

Although the structural basis of cancer networks is measured by 'The Manual', there is no coherent machinery for measuring the *implementation* of standards using *process and outcome* data. A series of clinical decisions is made for individual patients as they progress the 'patient journey'. However, such decisions can be based only on data available at that point. Data may be inaccurate or missing. There is currently no contractual obligation on clinicians in the NHS to ensure that clinicians complete a nationally agreed data-set in an *accurate and timely* fashion.

In summary, the following multiple data-sets are required for managed cancer networks in England:

* *The Manual of Cancer Service Standards* (NHS Executive 2001) governs the collection of data regarding *structures* (staffing and policies). A planned bi-annual

review of performance using 'The Manual' is likely to include measures of *implementation* of policies.

• The Gillis Report (2000) recommends the transfer of accountability for collecting the cancer registry core data-set to NHS trusts from 2001. This data-set currently includes *processes* such as pathological and radiological staging and treatment. Ultimately cancer registries link these data to epidemiological *outcome* measures such as mortality.

Other *processes* covering performance such as waiting times to treatment are collected through trust and health authority management systems. *The Cancer Minimum Dataset* (NHS Information Authority 2001) is designed to collect a series of *processes* for all patients with cancer.

From time to time, clinicians collect *retrospective* audit or *prospective* randomised clinical trial *outcome* data. These link individual patient survival times, response, recurrence and adverse events to individual treatment.

An external review of cancer data collection in the Kent Cancer Network identified a series of issues. These included:

• Difficulty in identifying cancer information and communication technology (ICT) leads in each trust.
• Data collection: duplication, missing fields, led by technology rather than strategy, lack of clarity over aims, uncertainty of who is responsible for corrective action.
• Management misunderstanding of professional needs/professional misunderstanding of management needs.
• Ignorance of 'network' approach to information strategy, including: a need for a centralised policy, cancer commissioning and budgetary control systems, forthcoming performance assessment and evidence-based protocols, network principles such as the 'patient journey'.
• Much discussion had taken place around technological developments, such as the need for a web-based booking and information system, but little on the practicalities of logging accurate data.

## Computer support for MDTs

Although the NHS has indicated its aspirations for the development of ICT support for the first decade of the twenty-first century (NHS 1998), and also published an information strategy document for cancer services (NHS 2000), the lesson of the past is that a monolithic ICT solution is not practical, and current activity is centred on a range of demonstrator projects (Bellingham 2001). A computer-based system to support MGTs would be in accord with this approach.

The particular areas of computer science that will inform the development of appropriate systems are studies of human–computer interface and computer-supported co-operative work. The basic aims of a computer-based system to support MDTs are to:

- collate and share data between team members
- allow data to be corrected if necessary
- record data for registry and other purposes
- record decisions
- record responsibilities contributing to and arising from the decisions
- provide a means for individuals to record their acknowledgements.

Achieving these aims will be no simple task. However, if, as seems highly probable, there will be a need to allow team members to participate in meetings by telephone, on-line computer or some other means, this will complicate the supporting computer-based system, and the need for reliable attribution is yet a further complication. These complications are not, however, unique to medical systems and there is scope to learn from other application areas. What follows is an account of experimental work that has implications for the design of a system to support MDTs. After a brief discussion of professional teams, the literature on systems supporting teams whose members may be in different places, or who may not all be free to attend meetings at the same time, is reviewed. Finally, the problem of accountability is discussed.

## Professional teams

Multidisciplinary teams in a cancer service, as in any other setting, need to work towards a common goal, and they need to be able to discuss differing views in a constructive manner. However, the orientation of professionals to competitive and individualistic attitudes, resulting in part from education, can frustrate this requirement. The professional norms of collegiality and equality can become translated into impersonal relationships where interpersonal difficulties and frictions are smoothed over, and where individuals focus on getting their own way. In studies of hospital management in the USA, Tjorvold and Tjorvold (1995) used interviews to establish factors which in turn established the distinctive role of shared goals and constructive controversy. The interviewees, nurse managers and physicians associated these with 'developing a shared purpose', 'understanding how their roles are interconnected', 'having a common task to complete' and 'seeing that they will be rewarded together'. These factors are primarily organisational and managerial; however, they may well be the significant determinant of the success or failure of the introduction of a computer-supported co-operative work system.

## Geographically dispersed teams

The reorganisation of cancer services as networks directly leads to the possibility of team meetings involving participants who may not all be in the same place. Although there is evidence that face-to-face meetings are more effective and preferred by participants (Straus 1997), there are obvious advantages to be gained by saving staff time and avoiding other costs associated with travel to participate in meetings. Research on computer systems to support mutually distant team members involved in collaborative work goes back several years, and Olson and Olson (2000) have reviewed the use of several systems of varying levels of technological sophistication. The systems studied have included scientific collaboration and sales strategy meetings, but more typical of the bulk of studies during the last 10 years has been the study of design teams working on software or engineering projects. Several factors stand out as being relevant to the success or failure of the systems. These are the extent to which collaborators share *common ground*, the extent to which work is *closely* or *loosely coupled*, the degree of *readiness for collaboration* among team members and the extent to which collaborators are comfortable with the *technologies* that they need to utilise. These four factors are first discussed and them related to MDTs.

### Common ground

'Common ground refers to that knowledge that participants have in common, and that they are aware that they have in common' (Olson & Olson 2000). This knowledge encompasses obvious facts about a shared environment, facts that are elicited during the course of an interchange, and knowledge based on mutual, prior acquaintance. Where teams are physically collocated, it seems relatively easy to establish common ground. Mutual knowledge of a common setting, awareness of each other's momentary activity, and facial and gestural expression together provide a supportive base for interaction. In discussions in which some physically remote participants are linked by means of audio or video, Olson and Olson point out not that it is impossible to develop common ground, but that it is more difficult and less likely to be successful. Moreover, they claim that additional bandwidth and novel technologies, although generally beneficial, have not always been successful; and they recommend the use of physically collocated meeting to establish common ground, as a preparation for subsequent dispersed meetings.

### Coupling of work

The extent to which common ground is vital can depend on how closely team members need to work with each other, and this in turn depends on how loosely or how tightly their work is coupled. Based on analyses of software and engineering design teams, Olson and Olson's studies show the benefits to be derived from allocating work in a way that reflects the location of workers. Work requiring high levels of interaction between workers benefits from collation. Work that is not tightly coupled is suitable for non-collocated team members. They further report that, with dispersed teams, a stricter protocol for governing interaction is required than necessary for a collocated team. It is particularly important that communications are acknowledged and that there are very clear indications of who is responsible for future actions.

## Collaboration readiness

Without appropriate preparation, computer-mediated work sharing may well be unsuccessful. Olson and Olson quote a pathetic lament from one interviewee in a computer-supported co-operative team: 'I keep feeling I've missed a meeting where all this was explained.' They go on to assert that, without a culture of sharing and collaboration, and without a supportive organisational framework and incentives, success is problematic. They quote Orlikowski's (1992) study of the use of Lotus Notes in a consultancy organisation, in which consultants had avoided learning to use the technology because there was no account to which to bill their learning time.

## Technology readiness

People working over networks can be asked to make use of hardware and software technologies of varying degrees of sophistication, and the effectiveness of the technologies may depend on working habits. Email, for example, loses its utility unless reading emails becomes part of collaborators' work routines. But, as well as reading emails, team members have to learn the complementary habit of making information available to their collaborators. The acquisition of such habits may take time, and so it can be advantageous only gradually to introduce the technology required to support dispersed groups.

The four factors discussed in the preceding sections need to be reflected on in the context of MDTs. There are likely to be good opportunities in managed care networks for team members to establish a fair degree of common ground at preparatory or other meetings; this could, in part, compensate for difficulties that might be encountered by participants in non-collocated team meetings.

The assessment activities of the members of MDTs are not likely to be tightly coupled as a result of the distinct professional orientation of team members. Their contributions stem from their professional backgrounds, which tend not to overlap. So, on this score, there is no reason to expect difficulties arising as a result of dependencies between team members. As for collaboration readiness and technology readiness, it depends on local circumstances. If the team members are prepared in both respects, there is nothing in the computer science literature that would predict that MDTs would not benefit from computer-supported non-collocated meetings.

## Group decision support systems and asynchronous support

Work by Nunamaker (1997), who has been an advocate of group decision support systems for several years, makes a strong case for their utility based on time saving and the quality of the decisions arrived at. His early work focused on the design of purpose-built computer-equipped rooms for collocated teams of decision-makers. In these rooms, each team member is allocated a computer and all team members can see and write to an additional wall-mounted display screen. Team members can simultaneously express their ideas by typing on their keyboards. These ideas may then be displayed on the shared display. Team members can also use their computers to access relevant data and software. The main advantage of such meetings over conventional meetings arises immediately from avoiding the time-wasting process of 'turn-taking' and by reducing the adverse effects on individual creativity of the inhibiting exposure to the presence of dominant personalities. Nunamaker points out other advantages stemming from 'anonymity, equal participation . . . and group memory capabilities that directly affect processes and outcomes'. His more recent work has been concerned with providing facilities for supporting teams separated by time and space, and he does not appear to share Olson and Olson's (2000) reservations about the inherent limitations of systems designed to mitigate the consequences of distance, nor does he share their awareness of the prerequisites for success. The use of virtual reality systems, which can provide a strong and vivid sense of presence of those unable to attend in person, is his favoured approach to supporting dispersed teams (Nunamaker 1997).

A rather different approach to group support systems is taken by Roseman and Greenberg (1996). Rather than design systems that concentrate on the notion of a 'meeting', their work exploits the metaphor of a 'place'. This means that their system, called TeamRooms, 'addresses the issue of what happens outside real-time collaboration'. This is achieved principally by providing easy and permanent access to shared documents. The interface for a TeamRoom is a web page, to which access is controlled by a central server. Among the facilities provided are:

- a simple text-based chat tool, which may be augmented by audio or video links
- a shared whiteboard with a range of different coloured pens
- a real-time video image of each currently active user
- a single cursor for each user that can be used to communicate simple pointing gestures
- a range of applets (small programs carried on a worldwide web page that can be activated by the viewer) providing application facilities such as databases and spreadsheets.

A claim that Roseman and Greenberg make, which is of particular interest for MDTs, is that TeamRooms greatly simplifies the set-up of real-time collaborations.

A commercial product called Teamwave Workplace has been developed (Greenberg 1999) and Greenberg has also been involved in the establishment of criteria for the selection of appropriate groupware products (Baker *et al*. 2001).

## Accountability and attribution

The traditional way of establishing accountabilities arising from decision-making meetings is the distribution and subsequent signing of minutes. This process may well be too leisurely and too broad to satisfy the requirements of MDTs. Decisions about the treatment of patients must be recorded so that:

• accurate data are collected,
• accountability for the accuracy of data is recorded
• responsibility for future action is clear to the participants and is also clearly recorded.

For the system designer, this does not require unfamiliar technology. The situation is similar to the recording of the details of a financial transaction. But there is, however, a possibility of conflict between, on the one hand, the need for effective collaboration, which is itself vital to medical outcomes and, on the other, legal accountability for individual decision and responsibility. This is reflected in analyses of error which take into account organisational factors as well as proximal actions (Reason 1990). In a paper that considers the concept of accountability both in a hospital radiology department and in connection with air traffic control, McCarthy *et al*. (1997) develop a framework that is relevant to designing a group decision support system for MDTs (in which the computer-based support might be but one of several elements). Its approach is to consider different aspects of the 'accountability for work activity', e.g. they distinguish between *explicit* and *implicit* accountability, where *explicit* refers to the use of externally verifiable procedures and specifications, and *implicit* refers to the range of unspecified practices that arise from the need to 'get things done'. They also discuss the complexities introduced by interdependencies of tasks within a job and how that can affect accountability. Their conclusion is that requirements analysis for high-consequence work systems must take into account the often subtle connections between accountability and work practices.

## Conclusion

Managed care networks require a novel approach to data collection and clinical governance, because decisions are corporate and clinical involvement might be via an electronic link. Prospective data collection requires *accountability* to be linked to *attributability* for data logging. Networks are more likely to involve transfer of patients *between* health sectors and *systemic* (multidisciplinary) rather than *individual* accountability. In NHS cancer networks, there is an urgent need to co-ordinate prospective data collection and clarify its relationship with clinical governance. At present a series of data-sets cover structural, process and outcome standards for cancer patients.

This chapter has discussed recent and current work on the use of computers to support co-operative group activities that are relevant to the development of systems for the support of MDTs. Although there are certainly accounts of systems that have successfully supported group decision-making, the general tenor of this literature is one of guarded optimism. Although distance still matters, much progress has been made in systems that compensate for team members not all being in the same place at the same time. Further, it is inevitable that networked computers will be used, to some extent, if only at a secretarial level, to support MDTs. The challenge ahead is to design ways of using computer-based systems that simultaneously accommodate the needs for data collection and accountability, but do not do so at the expense of medically correct and effective decision-making. Success will depend on a detailed understanding of the individual and group processes involved in decision-making, and a realistic assessment of the potentialities of current computing and communication technology.

## Recommendations

The collection of most *process-oriented* data for the three most common cancers should be via the MDT meeting held in most cancer units (hospitals) on a weekly basis.

Many data relevant to cancer are recorded on electronic systems in trust management, pathology or radiology departments. Research is needed to propose specification techniques for ICT systems to support MDT meetings or components of other relevant systems, and hence contribute to the incremental implementation of the 'Information for Health' agenda. There is also a need to show how data logging and attribution problems can be ameliorated through ICT-supported systems.

A coherent approach to clinical governance based on prospective data collection involves alignments with knowledge management, information systems specification and health informatics. It also implies the development of systems that will enable each health professional to co-operate in decision-making in such a way that decisions and commitments are attributable, and that quality assurance is facilitated to ensure that data collection is both accurate and timely.

*References*

Baker K, Greenberg S, Gutwin C (2001). Heuristic evaluation of groupware based on the mechanics of collaboration. Proceedings of the 8th IFIP Working Conference on Engineering for Human-Computer Interaction (EHCI'01), May 11–13, Toronto, Canada.

Bellingham A (2001). The Electronic Record: bringing it all together. Proceedings of conference 'Clinical Information Systems and Electronic Records 2001', London

Buckley G (1999). Revalidation is the answer. *British Medical Journal* **319**, 1145–1146

Clinical Standards Board for Scotland (2000). *Quality Assurance & Accreditation Manual*. Edinburgh: Clinical Standards Board for Scotland

Department of Health (1989). *Working for Patients*. Working Paper 6. London: HMSO

Department of Health (1995). *The Report of the Expert Advisory Group on Cancer to the Chief Medical Officers of England and Wales: a policy document for the commissioning of cancer services*. London: Department of Health, EL95(51)

The Gillis Report (2000). *Review of Cancer Registries in England*

Greenberg S (1999) The ebb and flow of collaboration in groupware. Invited plenary presentation. Proceedings of OZCHI'99 Australian conference on Human Computer Interaction, November 28–30, Wagga Wagga, Australia

McCarthy JC, Healey PGT, Wright PC, Harrison MD (1997) Accountability of work activity in high-consequence work systems: human error in context. International *Journal of Human-Computer Studies* **47**, 735–766

NHS (1998) *Information for Health 1998–2005*. London: HMSO

NHS (2000) *Cancer Information Strategy*. London: HMSO

NHS Executive (1999). *Faster Access to Modern Treatment: How NICE appraisal will work*. London: NHS Executive

NHS Executive (2001). *The Manual of Cancer Service Standards*. London: HMSO

NHS Information Authority (2001). *The Cancer Minimum Dataset*. London: HMSO

Nunamaker JF Jr (1997) Future research in group support systems: needs, some questions and possible directions. *International Journal of Human-Computer Studies* **47**, 357–385

Olson GM & Olson JS (2000). Distance matters. *Human Computer Interaction* **15**, 139–178

Orlikowski W (1992) Learning from Notes: Organizational issues in groupware implementation. Proceedings of the conference on computer supported cooperative work. ACM, pp 362–369

Reason J (1990) *Human Error*. Cambridge: Cambridge University Press

Roseman M & Greenberg S (1996) TeamRooms: networked places for collaboration. In Ackerman MS (ed.) *Proceedings, CSCW 96, ACM. Conference on computer supported cooperative work*. Cambridge, MA, pp. 325–333

Straus SG (1997) Technology, group process, and group outcomes: testing the connection in computer-mediated and face-to-face groups. *Human-Computer Interaction* **12**, 227–266

Tjorvold D & Tjorvold MM (1995). Cross-functional teamwork: the challenge of involving professionals. In Beyerlein MM, Johnson DA, Beyerlein ST (eds) *Advances in Interdisciplinary Studies of Work Teams: Knowledge work in teams*, Vol 2. Greenwich, CT: JAI Press, pp 1–34

# Index